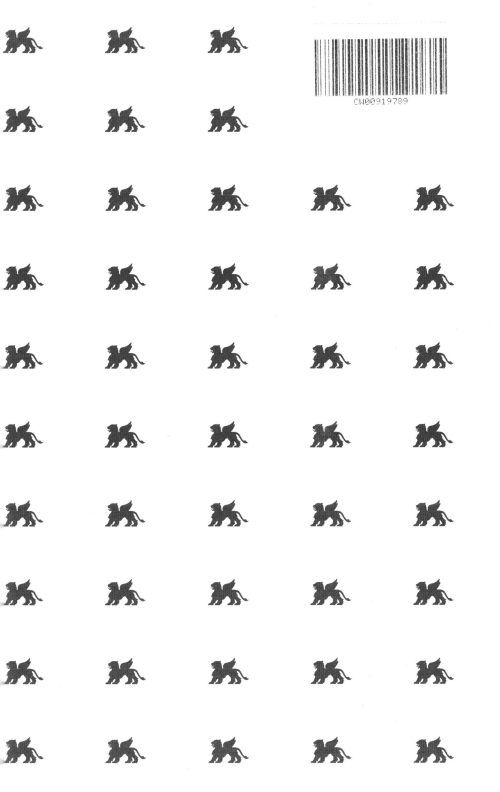

Stoma Care: A Guide for Patients

Rali Marinova

Petya Marinova

Zarah Perry-Woodford

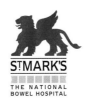

St MARK'S
THE NATIONAL
BOWEL HOSPITAL

Having a stoma may be overwhelming and challenging for you at first but your stoma nurse is here to guide and support you throughout your journey with a stoma.

Name	
Hospital number	
NHS Number	

Type of stoma	
Type of surgery	
Date of surgery	

Local stoma nurse	
St Mark's stoma nurses	Tel: 0208 453 2196 Email: LNWH-tr.stomacare@nhs.net Website: www.stmarkshospital.nhs.uk/stoma-care
Out of hours contact	Contact the ward from which you were discharged Call NHS 111 or visit 111.NHS.uk (for people aged 5 and over only) Attend your local emergency department
Consultant	

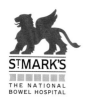

St MARK'S
THE NATIONAL
BOWEL HOSPITAL

©2021 St Mark's Academic Institute

All rights reserved. No part of this publication may be reproduced, distributed, or transmitted in any form or by any means, including photocopying, recording, or other electronic or mechanical methods, without the prior written permission of the publisher, except in the case of brief quotations embodied in critical reviews and certain other noncommercial uses permitted by copyright law. For permission requests, write to the publisher.

First published in the United Kingdom in 2021 by St Mark's Academic Institute, St Mark's Hospital, Central Middlesex Hospital, Acton Lane, Park Royal, London, NW10 7NS

Printed by Gwasg Gomer Cyf / Gomer Press Ltd, Parc Menter Llandysul, Llandysul, Ceredigion SA44 4JL.

Title: Stoma Care: A Guide for Patients

Authors: Rali Marinova, Petya Marinova, Zarah Perry-Woodford

Diagrams produced by Rali Marinova & Petya Marinova

Typesetting and design: Stephen Preston

ISBN: 978-0-9935363-3-5

Appendices

Glossary

References

Foreword

A stoma can be associated with both fear and prejudice. Much of this is generated by lack of information which can cause undue anxiety for many. It is not only the fear of the unknown but also how an individual will be accepted with a stoma. Appropriate information and support is key to ensuring that anyone needing a stoma has the smoothest journey.

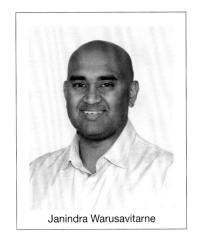

Janindra Warusavitarne

It has been an honour to be the Surgical Lead for stoma care at St Mark's Hospital and watch this world-class department grow even further under the expert leadership of Zarah Perry-Woodford, Consultant Nurse in stoma care.

This book is the testament to the world-class department and its quest to ensure that all patients with a stoma and those who may require a stoma, have contemporary, evidence-based information and I congratulate Rali and Petya Marinova for this important work. This book will offer all patients the information needed to dispel myths and attempt to allay any anxieties. Most importantly after reading this book the excellent stoma care team at St Mark's Hospital will be ready to answer any questions and offer all support needed.

Janindra Warusavitarne (B Med FRACS PhD)

Consultant Surgeon and Surgical Lead for Stoma Care

Introduction

A stoma should not prevent you from regaining the lifestyle you enjoyed before your operation, even though there will be some physical and emotional challenges to overcome along the journey. For many people a stoma can be freedom from the pain and uncertainty of living with a long-term illness. Regardless of the reason for stoma-forming surgery, most people become overwhelmed when sourcing, understanding or sharing the vast amount of available information.

The aim of this book is to reinforce what you have been told by the surgeon and stoma nurse prior to your surgery, signpost you to independently care for your stoma, make important decisions about your health and become confident in preventing and treating possible stoma complications. Moreover, this book will assist you in deciding whether it is safe to manage your stoma related problems on your own or seek help from a healthcare professional. We hope with guidance from your stoma nurse and this book, you will be able to incorporate your stoma into your life fairly quickly.

In this book we have used the symbols below to either highlight important information or direct you to other sections in the book where a full explanation is provided:

    very important information that should not be ignored

    specific information to St Mark's Hospital and not necessarily the advice of other colorectal hospitals or stoma nurses

    information that is documented in greater detail in either the '**general stoma care**' or '**complications related to stoma formation**' sections

The glossary at the end of this book provides an explanation of some of the medical terms and uncommon words used.

We would like to take this opportunity to thank our stoma nursing colleagues at St Mark's Hospital and NHS Supply Chain: Rehabilitation, Disabled Services, Women's Health and Associated Consumables Provided by Collaborative Procurement Partnership, for their continuous motivation and support in allowing us time to write this book. Additionally, we are grateful for the guidance from Mr Janindra Warusavitarne, Professor Sue Clark and Mr Stephen Preston for their editorial input and expertise.

Special thanks to our past patients for providing the written testimonials and to members of the InsideOut Stoma Support Group, for taking the time to critique the contents within.

We would like to express our sincere gratitude to Dansac Ltd and InsideOut for their financial support in publishing this book and for their investment in supporting our patients.

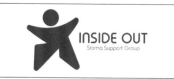

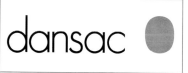

This is a non-profit book and it relies on donations. If you would like to help fund reprinting and distribution of this book, you can make a donation by using a Direct Debit or Online Banking. When making a donation please remember to quote **'Stoma book'** as payment reference.

Account Name: St Mark's Hospital Foundation

Account Number: 00085102

Sort Code: 40-52-40

This book is dedicated to the memory of Joachim (Joe) Dyer (1977–2017) who battled the challenges of stoma care in the most dignified and determined manner. He is the inspiration for this book and the hope that the information helps others on their journey with a stoma.

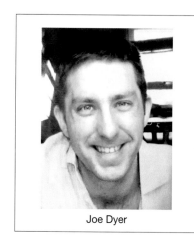

Joe Dyer

Biography

Rali Marinova (RGN, BSc, MSc)

Having qualified as a nurse in 2016, I moved to Ireland where I worked on a surgical ward. After moving to the UK in 2018 to work as a nurse on a urology ward in London, I then joined St Mark's Hospital working on the colorectal ward in 2019. Later that year I joined the Stoma Care team where I have been working as a Specialist Stoma Nurse. I have gained great experience in looking after stoma and enterocutaneous fistulae patients on both acute wards and in nurse-led stoma care clinics, as well as, participating in research, department audits, protocols development and in-house staff education.

Petya Marinova (RGN, BSc, MSc)

I qualified as a nurse in 2016 and shortly after that moved to Ireland where I worked on a general surgery and colorectal ward. Then, in 2018 I moved to the UK to work as a nurse on a urology ward in London. In 2019, I joined St Mark's Hospital working on the colorectal ward. Later that year I joined the Stoma Care department team where I have been working as a Specialist Pouch Nurse. While working in the Internal Pouch Care team, I have gained great experience in looking after pouch, stoma and enterocutaneous fistulae patients on both acute wards and in nurse-led stoma care clinics, as well as, participating in research, department audits, protocols development and in-house staff education.

Zarah Perry-Woodford (RGN, MSc, Non-Medical Prescriber)

I have been a nurse for over 24 years with 20 years in the field of colorectal surgery and stoma care. My first nursing role was as a military nurse serving in the Royal Air Force. In 2002, I joined St Mark's Hospital in London, working as a Senior Staff Nurse on the colorectal ward before joining the stoma team as a Specialist Nurse, managing patients with stomas, ileoanal pouches, enterocutaneous fistulae and those requiring intestinal rehabilitation. I spent 12 years developing and expanding the current ileoanal pouch service running nurse-led clinics and an email and telephone advice line. In 2018, I became a Consultant Nurse, where I remain dedicated to contributing to pre and post graduate nurse education by supporting current research/protocol development, publishing in a variety of medical and nursing journals and presenting at national and international conferences.

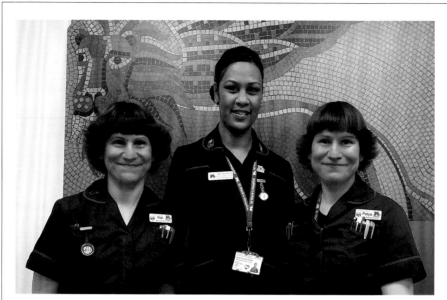

Rali Marinova, Zarah Perry-Woodford, Petya Marinova

1. Preparing for surgery

Digestive and urinary systems

Digestive system (gastrointestinal tract) – is a complex system made up of both hollow (tube-like) and solid organs, with various functions. The hollow organs include your mouth, oesophagus (gullet or food pipe), stomach, gallbladder, small intestine, large intestine (colon), rectum and anus. The solid organs include the liver and pancreas.

The role of your digestive system is to:

- digest the food and fluids you eat and drink

- absorb water, nutrients, minerals and vitamins

- eliminate waste products

Digestion starts in your mouth, which is why it is very important to chew your food well. Once your food is swallowed, it travels down your oesophagus until it reaches your stomach, where it continues to be digested, as it moves along to your intestines.

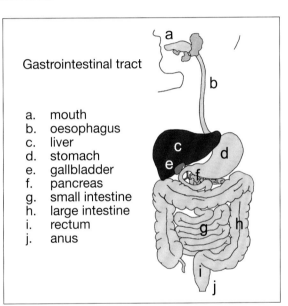

Gastrointestinal tract

a. mouth
b. oesophagus
c. liver
d. stomach
e. gallbladder
f. pancreas
g. small intestine
h. large intestine
i. rectum
j. anus

Small intestine – is approximately **6.5 m long** and includes the duodenum, jejunum and ileum. Its main function is to absorb nutrients. As food and fluid travel down your small intestine, **water, nutrients, minerals and vitamins are gradually absorbed** and the intestinal content becomes thicker. Hence, the further along the small intestine a stoma is formed, the more water and electrolytes will be absorbed and the stoma output will be less watery.

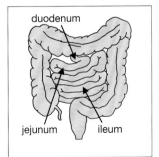

The **duodenum** is the first part of the small intestine (about 25 cm long). This is where secretions from pancreas and gallbladder help break down the food.

The **jejunum** is the upper two–fifths of the small intestine (about 2.5 m long). This is where further protein, fats and carbohydrates are digested.

The **ileum** is the lower three–fifths of the small intestine (about 3.6 m long). This is where the body absorbs glucose and sodium. The last part of the ileum (terminal ileum) is responsible for vitamin B_{12} absorption.

Large intestine (colon) – is about **1.5 m long** and consists of the appendix, caecum, ascending colon, transverse colon, descending colon, sigmoid colon, rectum and anus. Its main functions are further **water and electrolyte absorption and elimination of waste products.** Synthesis of vitamin K and some B–complex vitamins also occur in

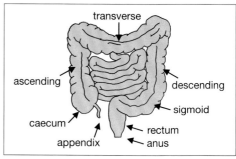

the colon. Every day the colon absorbs about 1–2 litres of water with most of this occurring in the caecum and in the ascending colon. As food and fluids travel down your large intestine, water, nutrients, minerals, and vitamins are gradually absorbed and the intestinal content gets thicker. At the time of evacuation, approximately 100–200 ml of solid stool is passed.

Urinary system – consists of two kidneys, two ureters, the bladder and urethra. The function of the urinary tract is to:

- transport and store urine

- remove waste products

- regulate fluid and electrolyte balance

- regulate acid–base balance in your body

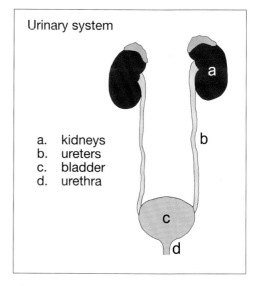

Urinary system

a. kidneys
b. ureters
c. bladder
d. urethra

Kidneys – most people have two kidneys. Each kidney is located on either side at the back of your body, just below your ribs. Their function is to control our body water content, minerals composition and acidity. The kidneys also metabolise vitamin D, control sodium level, produce urine and eliminate waste products from your body.

Ureters – most people have two ureters. They look like little tubes starting from your kidney and ending at the base of your bladder, carrying urine from the kidney.

Bladder – the bladder stores urine. Usually when the urine volume in your bladder reaches around 200–400 ml, the need to pass urine is felt.

Urethra – the urethra transports urine from your bladder to outside your body, as you pass urine. Female urethras are approximately 4–5 cm long, while male urethras are significantly longer, approximately 20 cm.

What is a stoma?

A stoma is a surgically created opening into the abdomen which is used to divert the flow of faeces or urine (stoma output) outside the body. The intestine (bowel) is brought up through this opening and stitched to the skin. The peristomal skin (area around the stoma) can be easily damaged by the stoma output due to the disturbance of the natural pH of the skin in the presence of urine, faeces or digestive enzymes. It is, therefore, vital stoma care is understood and practised effectively.

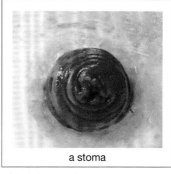
a stoma

The expelled stoma output is collected in a bag which is stuck on your abdomen called **a stoma bag, pouching system or appliance**.

There are several types of stomas which differ according to what is expelled from the stoma or which part of the intestine is used to create the stoma. The stoma types discussed in this book are **ileostomy, colostomy, urostomy and jejunostomy**. A stoma may be either permanent or temporary, however, a urostomy is always permanent. A permanent stoma will not be reversed, while a temporary stoma can be reversed within 3–12 months or longer, depending on your general health and recovery after surgery.

☐ Ileostomy

An ileostomy is formed from the lower part of your small intestine (ileum). Since the contents do not enter the large intestine, some of the water, salt and nutrients that used to be absorbed in the large intestine, will be lost through the ileostomy.

Bile and pancreatic juice are secreted into the small intestine to aid with digestion, therefore, the output from an ileostomy will always be a semi-liquid (porridge-like) or liquid consistency.

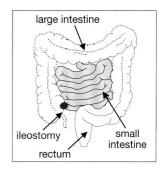
large intestine

ileostomy
rectum
small intestine

Colostomy

A colostomy is formed from part of your large intestine (colon). Since you still have most of your large intestine, it will continue to absorb the majority of the water, salt and nutrients.

Therefore, the output from a colostomy will usually be of a semi-formed or solid consistency. Occasionally due to infection or changes in diet or medication, the output may become more liquid.

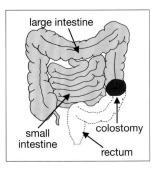

Urostomy (ileal-conduit)

A urostomy is formed using 15–25 cm of your small intestine which is surgically removed from your digestive system. Your ureters will be detached from the bladder (which is then removed) and attached to the piece of small intestine. This is referred to as an ileal-conduit. The ileal-conduit is brought up through the abdomen to skin level and stitched to the skin, and is now referred to as the urostomy. Urine from the kidneys will travel through the ileal-conduit, before exiting the abdomen via the urostomy. The role of the intestine will not be affected and therefore your bowel function remains the same.

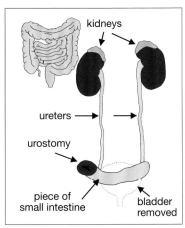

Jejunostomy

A jejunostomy is formed from the middle part of your small intestine (jejunum). Since your large intestine and most of your small intestine do not take part in the digestion anymore, large volumes of water, salt and nutrients will be lost through your jejunostomy. Therefore, your output will be of a liquid consistency, high volume and contain a high concentration of salt and nutrients.

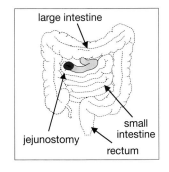

Mucous fistula

A mucous fistula is formed when either an ileostomy or a colostomy is created and the rectum is left in place. The top end of the rectum may be surgically closed and remains inside your abdomen or it may be left open and brought onto the surface of the skin as a mucous fistula. A mucous fistula may be positioned just below your ileostomy or colostomy or at any other location on the abdomen. The mucous fistula does not produce any faeces only mucus, which is the lubricant produced by your intestine to aid the passage of faeces. The mucus may pass either through the mucous fistula or through the anus. If the mucous fistula is positioned directly below your ileostomy or colostomy, you will need to cut a slightly larger hole in the stoma bag, to

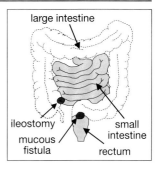

allow the mucus to drain into the stoma bag. However, if your mucous fistula is positioned away from your stoma, you will need to use a different stoma appliance known as a **stoma cap**.

Stoma configurations

A stoma may be formed as an end, loop or double-barrel configuration.

End stoma

Formed from the end of your intestine or when only **one** end or opening is brought out to skin level. The other end may have been removed or surgically closed and left inside the abdomen.

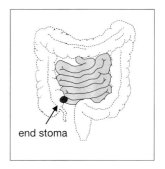

Loop stoma

A **loop** of your intestine is brought out through the abdominal wall and then partially cut, the edges folded back and stitched to the skin, forming two stoma openings, one from the upper part of your intestine (proximal stoma) and the other one from the lower part (distal stoma). The proximal loop will produce output, while the distal loop is excluded from the digestive process. The distal

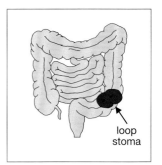

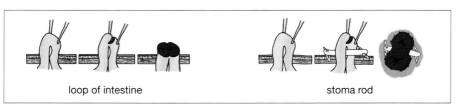

loop still produces mucus which may be visible when changing the stoma bag.

A loop stoma is usually temporary and mainly formed in cases when a section of diseased intestine has been removed and the healthy intestine is then joined together (an anastomosis). The anastomosis needs to be protected, therefore, the loop stoma is fashioned above the join allowing the intestine below the stoma to heal. In some cases, if your surgeon thinks there may be too much tension on your intestine when creating your stoma, a small plastic rod/bridge may be placed underneath the loop of intestine to ensure the stoma does not retract below skin level. The rod sits on your abdomen and after 3–5 days will be removed by your stoma nurse or surgeon. Having a rod/bridge may make your stoma care training a bit more complex at first, but it should not delay your discharge, as your stoma nurse will still be able to train you on how to care for your stoma.

Double-barrel stoma

Similar to a loop stoma, but instead of having a loop of intestine, a double-barrel stoma has **two separate ends** of intestine brought out through the abdominal wall, forming two separate stomas. One stoma produces faecal output, while the other stoma will only produce mucus. In most cases both the small intestine and large intestine are used to create the double-barrel stoma.

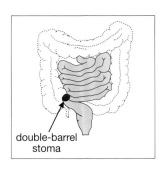

double-barrel stoma

Indications for stoma formation

In the UK, there are over 205,000 children and adults[1] with a stoma (ostomates) with approximately 25,000 new stomas[2] formed each year. The main reasons for stoma formation is to:

- protect a surgical join in the intestine
- divert the faeces or urine when an area of intestine or bladder is removed
- divert the intestine above a significant stricture, obstruction or tear
- prevent faecal or urinary contamination in the abdomen
- allow intestinal healing

There are various diseases or conditions which require stoma formation, the most common are:

☐ **Cancer**

If you have cancer involving your small or large intestine, then you may require a stoma. Intestinal cancer does not automatically mean that you will need a stoma but the stoma nurse may be asked to prepare you in case a stoma is required. Whether or not you require a stoma will depend on many factors, such as the exact location of your cancer, how advanced your disease is, if other organs are involved, whether or not you may need to have chemotherapy or radiotherapy after surgery and the opinion of your surgeon, oncologist and other experts involved in your treatment.

If you have a urinary tract or bladder cancer, a urostomy may be formed. In some cases if the cancer has penetrated the intestine and bladder you may require both an intestinal and urinary stoma.

☐ **Crohn's disease**

Crohn's disease is an inflammatory bowel disease (IBD) that may affect any part of your digestive tract. The lesions caused by the inflammation tend to skip certain areas but are commonly found at the end of the small intestine called the **terminal ileum**. The cause of Crohn's disease is usually related to an abnormal immune response and genetics, even though it is not clear what exactly triggers the disease. First degree relatives (mother, father, sister or brother) of patients with IBD are more likely to develop Crohn's disease, in comparison to the general population.

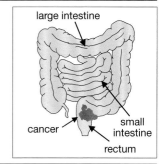

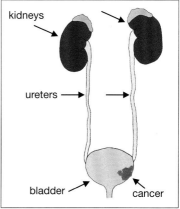

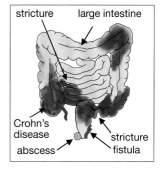

The most common signs and symptoms of Crohn's disease are:

- frequent and urgent bowel motions with bloody diarrhoea
- abdominal pain and cramping
- constipation
- weight loss
- abscesses
- fissures (small tears in the lining of the anus, which can be extremely

painful)

- fistulae (abnormal formation of a tunnel between two hollow organs or one hollow organ and the surface of the skin)
- intestinal strictures (abnormal narrowing of your intestine)

Most patients can be managed by medical treatment long term, however, if complications such as excessive bleeding, fistula formation, intestinal obstruction or perforation occur, surgery should be considered. The main types of operations performed for Crohn's disease are:

- bowel resection
- strictureplasty (surgical repair of abnormal narrowing of the intestine)

If a portion of your intestine needs to be removed, you may require a stoma which may either be temporary or permanent. Whether you require a stoma and for how long will depend on the progression of your disease, your general health and the opinion of your surgeon and gastroenterologist.

☐ Ulcerative colitis

Ulcerative colitis is a chronic condition. It is unknown what triggers the disease, but it is believed that it is a result of an overactive immune response. It is characterised by inflammation and ulceration within your rectum and large intestine. Symptoms may vary with or without treatment and this results in unpredictable periods of remission and relapse.

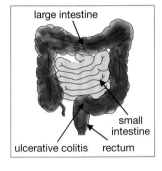

The most common signs and symptoms of ulcerative colitis are:

- frequent and urgent bowel motions with bloody diarrhoea
- abdominal pain and cramping
- blood and mucus in the faeces
- fever
- weight loss

Most patients can be managed successfully with medical treatments, but over time there is a chance of about a quarter to one third of people requiring an operation. The main types of surgery performed for ulcerative colitis are:

- subtotal colectomy and a temporary ileostomy
- panproctocolectomy and a permanent ileostomy

- restorative proctocolectomy with ileal pouch-anal anastomosis, with or without a temporary ileostomy
- ileorectal anastomosis – in this case, you will not have a stoma as the large intestine is removed and the small intestine joined to the rectum

Whether you require a stoma will depend on the progression of your disease, development of dysplasia or colonic cancer, your general health and the opinion of your surgeon and gastroenterologist.

Diverticular disease

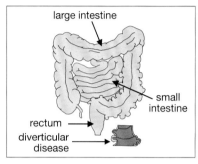

Diverticular disease is characterised by the formation of small pockets (diverticula) in the wall of your large intestine. These pockets could form anywhere in your large intestine, but most commonly in your sigmoid colon. The pockets can become blocked with faecal matter which then become inflamed. Inflammation of the pockets is called diverticulitis. Diverticulitis is usually treated with antibiotics and changes to your diet or lifestyle. However, in some cases the inflammation may become more serious and cause a perforation (tear) of the large intestine. In cases of perforation or repeating diverticulitis, your surgeon will remove the portion of diseased large intestine and you may require stoma formation. The decision will be based on your general health and the opinion of your surgeon.

Polyposis

Most bowel cancers develop from precancerous growths called polyps. In some cases, you may only have a few polyps, which are usually removed during a procedure called colonoscopy. In other cases, you may have numerous polyps inside your intestine called polyposis. Usually when there are too many polyps in your intestine the best option is to remove the area affected by polyposis. Your surgeon will decide whether it would be best to remove the diseased area and re-join the intestine or create a stoma.

Polyposis syndromes are often hereditary and passed on in your family. There are quite a few different types of polyposis syndromes, such as:

- Familial adenomatous polyposis (FAP)
- Peutz Jeghers syndrome (PJS)
- Juvenile polyposis syndrome (JPS)
- MYH associated polyposis (MAP)

- Serrated polyposis syndrome (SPS)
- Lynch syndrome

The Polyposis Registry based at St Mark's Hospital in London, represents one of the longest running research projects in the world (established in 1924). The Polyposis Registry contains information on over 3000 families with hereditary polyposis and allows families to be screened or followed up with regular endoscopy in order to detect signs for early surgical review.

The Wolfson Unit for Endoscopy at St Mark's Hospital is also world-renowned, having developed regional and national referral services for polypectomy, video capsule endoscopy and double-balloon enteroscopy, as well as providing nationally accredited courses for the training of endoscopists.

☐ Ischaemic bowel

Your intestine needs a blood supply to provide vital oxygen in order to function. If the blood supply is limited or stopped altogether, your intestine could become ischaemic. Prolonged ischaemia causes the intestine to become necrotic (cell death). Necrosis is a very serious condition and needs to be treated immediately. If you develop an ischaemic bowel your surgeon may need to remove a portion of your damaged intestine and you may require stoma formation.

The reasons for ischaemic bowel vary but the most common causes are:

- blocked artery – a blood clot in an artery supplying either your large or small intestine will limit the blood supply to your intestine. Depending on the severity of the blocked artery, a portion of your intestine may become necrotic.
- volvulus – abnormal twisting of your intestine, which could restrict blood flow.
- hernia – a portion of your intestine may slip through the hernia opening and become trapped, therefore, the blood flow to your intestine may become restricted.
- tumour – a large tumour will expand the walls of your intestine and may restrict the blood flow.
- recreational drugs – such as cocaine or methamphetamine can reduce blood flow to the intestine leading to ischaemia and necrosis over time.
- vigorous exercise – such as long distance running, can make your body restrict blood flow to your intestine, as it needs to concentrate your blood supply to your heart and muscles, limiting the blood supply for your intestine, though this is a rare occurrence.

☐ Trauma

Road traffic accidents, crush injuries, gunshot or stab wounds which damage either your urinary tract or intestine may require surgery in order to divert urine or faeces away from the damaged portion of your bladder or intestine and allow healing.

You will most likely require a temporary stoma, however if irreversible damage has been done, then your stoma will be permanent.

☐ Incontinence

If you have difficulty with either controlling your bowel movements or passing urine, you have a condition known as incontinence. Incontinence could be either faecal, urinary or both. The reasons for people to become incontinent are various. Some of the most common reasons for incontinence are:

- natural ageing process
- multiple pregnancies
- injury to your pelvic floor or sphincter muscles during childbirth
- spinal cord injury
- progressive neurodegenerative disorders such as Parkinson's disease and multiple sclerosis
- trauma

Some people choose to manage incontinence problems conservatively with incontinence pads or medication. However, if this is not an acceptable option for you and your surgeon considers it appropriate, you could opt for stoma-forming surgery in order to manage your incontinence and improve your quality of life.

☐ Intestinal perforation (tear)

Your intestine may become perforated for reasons such as disease progression, abdominal trauma or long-term use of some medications or recreational drugs. Perforation usually results in emergency surgery and stoma formation.

☐ Intestinal stricture

Your intestine may develop strictures (narrowing) for reasons such as disease progression or scar tissue formation following surgery. A stricture may make passage of intestinal content difficult and lead to bowel obstruction. You will need an operation to remove the portion of intestine with the stricture and in some cases a temporary stoma may be formed.

☐ **Congenital disorder (birth defect)**

A temporary stoma may be created until the new-born is old enough for corrective surgery of the defect.

Role of the stoma nurse

The stoma nurses at St Mark's Hospital are trained to care for stoma patients during their entire journey with a stoma. Your stoma nurse will be there to answer all your questions and help you adjust to life with a stoma, before your stoma-forming surgery, during your hospital stay and after your discharge home. St Mark's Hospital is a national centre of excellence and a world-renowned hospital for colorectal disease. The stoma nurses who work here are highly skilled and experienced nurses who regularly participate in stoma related audit, research and development in order to provide you with high quality, evidence-based care. We support both nursing and medical staff in order to maintain and improve standards of stoma care at national and international levels, however, some of our best lessons are learnt through supporting our patients or working with members from our stoma support groups and charities.

St Mark's Hospital stoma care vision and mission statement

Vision: To make certain every patient undergoing stoma-forming surgery is well supported, understood and empowered to ensure optimal quality of life is restored.

Mission Statement: The stoma care department at St Mark's Hospital is dedicated to providing individualised, expert and research-based nursing care within the field of colorectal surgery. We aim to offer sustainable services for both inpatients and outpatients, providing an exceptional experience for all.

For our patients and our community we aim to:

- treat all patients with dignity and respect.
- provide high quality, evidence-based clinical care.
- select appropriate and economical yet high quality stoma appliances and accessories that allow patients to return to the lifestyle they desire.
- form effective partnerships with the multi-disciplinary teams both locally and nationally in order to provide a seamless transfer for patients from acute hospital services into community care.
- develop robust links with patients to offer long-term support and review.
- continue to develop and support nursing/medical staff in order to maintain and improve standards of care in line with the Trust, the

Nursing and Midwifery Council and national stoma care guidelines.

Before your operation

When your surgeon has explained the best operation for your condition, they will refer you to a stoma nurse who will see you in an outpatient clinic. During your first meeting, your stoma nurse will go into detail about the type of stoma you will have which relates to the type of operation agreed for your treatment. You will also receive a huge amount of information, most of which is incorporated in this book, as we understand that you may not be able to take it all in. If it is too overwhelming to see us immediately after seeing the surgeon, we may give you this book to read, our contact details and then make another appointment for you to see us before your operation.

Topics covered by your stoma nurse:

- explanation of the surgical procedure and lifestyle implications
- type of stoma you will have
- choosing the best site on your abdomen for your stoma (stoma siting)
- explanation of the different types of stoma bags
- recovery from surgery
- stoma management
- diet
- lifestyle
- long-term stoma care, complication prevention and management
- ongoing delivery of stoma products
- returning to work
- travel
- sexuality and body image
- managing expectations
- psycho-social support

Stoma siting – once your stoma nurse discusses the topics mentioned above and you have been given an operation date, they will mark the best possible site on your abdomen for your stoma to be formed.

Choosing the most appropriate site for your stoma is very important, as this would make it easier for you to manage your stoma and return to your life as soon as possible post-surgery. Your stoma nurse will always consider your lifestyle and try to accommodate your preferences but sometimes you may not like the position your stoma nurse considers best for you.

Some compromises may need to be made, as they will also have to use their clinical judgement and medical knowledge, in order to ensure a safe position for your stoma is selected.

When choosing the best stoma site for you, any **scars, bony areas, the midline of your abdomen, umbilicus (belly button), belt line, skin folds, creases and dips** are avoided, as those may prevent your stoma appliance from achieving a good seal and cause leaks. However, if any of those situations are unavoidable, your stoma nurse may discuss your options with a colleague or the surgical team to ensure you have the most appropriate stoma site.

The shape of your abdomen changes when you move, so during the siting procedure you will be asked to **lie down, sit, stand, and bend forward** with your abdomen exposed, in order for your stoma nurse to observe for any scars, skin folds or creases that could cause problems once the stoma is formed. You would also be asked to cough or sit up as this helps detect your abdominal muscles. If the stoma is placed within a strong abdominal muscle (rectus sheath) this will offer support for your stoma and possibly reduce the risk of ☐ hernia and ☐ prolapse formation. Deep skin creases may be marked with a permanent marker pen so it is clear to your surgeon that there are creases to be avoided, in case your stoma site needs to be altered during surgery. Your surgeon will usually use the stoma mark selected by your stoma nurse and will only move it if it is absolutely necessary to do so during surgery.

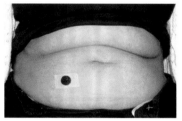

The initial mark will be placed on a piece of tape at first so it can be moved around, until the correct position is found.

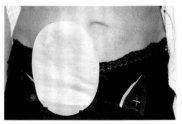

A stoma bag will be placed on your abdomen to make sure the stoma mark is at the most appropriate position.

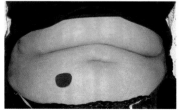

The final site is marked with a permanent marker pen and covered with a waterproof dressing.

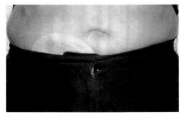

If your waistband is low the stoma bag will usually be visible over your belt line.

Your stoma nurse will question you about your lifestyle, religion, clothing, work and recreational activities. These questions not only help determine which site will be best for your stoma to be formed at but also help with discharge planning when you leave hospital. Whether you wear a belt or braces will be taken into consideration, so you do not necessarily have to change the way you dress just because you have a stoma. Your belt line is avoided as much as possible. Your stoma site would ideally be either above or below your belt line but unfortunately the safest place may be on your current belt line. Once your stoma site has been chosen, your stoma nurse will mark it with a permanent marker pen and cover it with a dressing. **In some cases two stomas are required and the process will be repeated to ensure both sites are ideal**.

In more complex cases, you may be marked on both sides of your abdomen or be given a higher and lower site on the same side of your abdomen. This gives the surgeon options, which allow them to still place the stoma in a suitable position if the first site is not safe to use during the operation. **However, being marked twice in this case does not mean that you will have two stomas**. The preferred site will be documented in your notes and discussed with the surgeon.

You will be given the marker pen and spare dressings to take home with you to use over your stoma site in case you notice it is fading. Once the ideal site for your stoma has been agreed, you will be asked to sign a consent form acknowledging that you understand the reasons for your stoma position.

You may also be given a small stoma kit to take home, so you can practise using your measuring guide, cutting the stoma bags and if you feel confident, attaching your stoma bag on your abdomen. This will give you an opportunity to become more familiar with what it will be like to have a stoma. Care must be taken removing the stoma bag especially if you have already been sited for your stoma as you do not want to remove the mark.

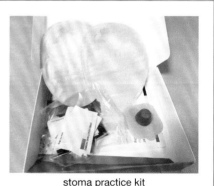

stoma practice kit

Surgical options

Your surgeon will explain which operation is most suitable for you as there are certain criteria for your chosen operation. For example, if you previously had open surgery, you may not be a suitable candidate for laparoscopic or robotic surgery. The main types of operations are:

Laparotomy (open surgery) – involves making a large midline incision (cut) to your abdomen to remove the disease and to form your stoma. Typically patients are expected to be in hospital for 10–14 days.

Laparoscopic (keyhole) – during laparoscopic surgery, your surgeon makes small cuts (port sites) on your abdomen to allow the insertion of various instruments to remove the diseased intestine and to form your stoma. The diseased intestine is then removed through a larger incision or the stoma site.

Robotic surgery – uses a highly advanced surgical robot to hold the instruments required in the operation and is controlled by the surgeon using a computer system rather than holding the instruments themselves.

Sometimes it may be necessary to change to open surgery (laparotomy) from laparoscopic or robotic surgery, if the procedure becomes technically difficult, as it is safer for you.

Enhanced recovery after surgery (ERAS)

St Mark's Hospital offers an ERAS programme for laparoscopic, robotic and some selected open surgery patients, but depends greatly on your general health, active participation post-surgery and ability to self-care. Discharge from hospital after ERAS is expected within 3–4 days post-surgery. The programme is based on a combination of interventions that have been researched and shown to improve patient outcomes and reduce hospital stay. Most patients are included in the ERAS programme, however, patients requiring more complex surgery may not be suitable candidates and follow a traditional recovery programme.

Pre-assessment – before your admission you will be invited to come to the hospital for blood tests, an electrocardiogram (ECG) and X–ray scan as necessary. The pre-assessment nurses will provide you with detailed information regarding the ERAS pathway and it will be explained to you what your role is in your recovery. You may be advised to stop smoking and drinking alcohol, eat healthy or start exercising in the few weeks before your operation. Your stoma nurse may come to speak to you about your stoma, give you this book and a stoma practice kit to take home. If your operation is within a few weeks you may be sited for your stoma on the same day.

Preparing for your surgery – you may be asked to take a bowel preparation (laxative) in the afternoon before the day of your surgery. If you need to be admitted the day before your surgery, these laxatives will be given to you on the ward. If you are admitted on the day of surgery, you will need to take these laxatives at home.

If you need bowel preparation, you will also need to switch to low fibre/low residue diet two days before your surgery (**avoid** wholemeal foods, raw fruits and vegetables, nuts, seeds, mushrooms, red meat). Then from midday on the day before your surgery, you will need to switch to a liquid diet (black coffee, water, squash, juice, clear soup and jelly). If you do not need to have bowel preparation you can eat until midnight the night before or six hours before your surgery and then have clear fluids (black tea, black coffee, water and squash, **no drinks containing milk**) up to **two** hours before your surgery. If you have been diagnosed with a hiatus hernia or suffer with heartburn, you should stop having anything to drink **four** hours before your surgery.

You will also need to have a blood thinning injection to protect against clot formations, as you are at higher risk of blood clots while in hospital, during and after surgery. If you are admitted the day before your surgery, this injection will be given to you on the ward or be given to you during your pre-assessment appointment to do yourself at home on the day before your hospital admission.

Admission to hospital – you may either be admitted to hospital the day before your surgery or on the day of your surgery. Your doctors and nurses will admit you on the ward by completing your admission paperwork and placing identity bands around your wrists and ankles. Ward staff may take blood samples and may insert a needle in your arm or hand so that medications and fluids can be given to you if needed. You will be given a gown and stockings to wear before going to theatre. Stoma-forming surgery may take many hours to complete and you will also spend some time in the recovery unit, so it is worth informing your relatives that they should contact the ward first to find out when it is appropriate for you to have visitors. If your relatives are particularly concerned, the surgeon may be able to contact a nominated relative immediately after your operation to inform them of your condition.

If you have not had your stoma sited prior to coming into hospital, your stoma nurse will meet you on the ward and site you.

 In the unlikely event your stoma site has not been marked before going to theatre, inform the ward staff immediately and they will contact a stoma nurse to come and do this for you.

Day of surgery (before your operation) – you may be given two high carbohydrate drinks at around 5 or 6 o'clock in the morning before your operation. This will depend on what type of surgery you are having and whether or not your surgeon considers this appropriate for you. You may be allowed to drink clear fluids until two to four hours before your surgery. In some cases you may need to have an enema early in the morning to help clear the lower part of your intestine.

Day 0 (after your operation) – you will be taken to recovery or intensive care unit until you are stable enough to return to a ward. You will have a tube, called a urinary catheter, in your bladder to collect urine, as you will not be very mobile initially. You will also have an intravenous drip going through a vein in your arm, hand or neck, to help keep you hydrated and for administering necessary medication. It is important to keep you comfortable post-surgery, therefore, you will be given some form of pain relief. This could be done either through a patient controlled analgesia (PCA), which is delivered through the drip in your hand or arm and is controlled by you pressing a button when you need it, or an epidural catheter inserted in your back. You may have tubes (drains) coming out of your abdomen which prevent fluid collecting and cause an infection. If you feel nauseated or experience vomiting post-surgery you may have a tube inserted through your nose and going down your throat all the way to your stomach to relieve the pressure. If you can tolerate fluids you will be offered water and/or two high-protein drinks.

You may also have a sore throat due to the breathing tube inserted down your throat during surgery but this should resolve within a few days. Some people experience shoulder pain which is unique to laparoscopic surgery due to the phrenic nerve irritation to the diaphragm caused by the carbon dioxide gas left in the abdomen post-surgery. When you sit up, the gas moves upwards to the diaphragm and irritates the shoulder area but this is not of concern and will disappear in a couple of days. You will be assisted to sit on the edge of the bed or sit in a chair shortly after you wake up from surgery. Remember that your recovery time will depend a lot on your willingness to mobilise early rather than lie in bed.

Your stoma nurse may visit to check the stoma, offer you emotional support and deliver a wash bag with all the necessary products for your stoma care, such as stoma bags, pair of scissors, adhesive remover spray, pen, wipes, water bowl, rubbish bags, mirror and a measuring guide.

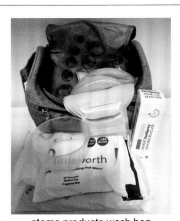

stoma products wash bag

This wash bag is yours to keep. If you are alert and able, you can observe the stoma bag being changed. You will be able to view your stoma as you will have a clear drainable bag on your abdomen to allow medical and nursing staff to monitor your stoma for possible complications.

Your stoma may seem quite swollen and big but this is completely normal and it will gradually become smaller over the next few weeks. You will also have stitches around your stoma which are used to anchor the stoma to your skin. The stitches will dissolve or fall out, usually within 3–4 weeks. Sometimes the stitches may be tucked up under the stoma so are not visible. A healthy stoma is moist and red in colour and raised above your skin. A clear bag would usually be used for the first 1–2 days after your operation and then be switched to an opaque bag that disguises your stoma and its output. Some people find it easier to continue to manage their stoma with a clear stoma bag and choose to be discharged home with one. You will initially have a one-piece stoma appliance but depending on your needs may benefit from a two-piece stoma appliance.

Stoma training and emotional support

At first you may think having a stoma is too overwhelming for you and begin to doubt your abilities to care for your stoma on your own. Most people with a new stoma initially feel this way and it is quite normal but your stoma nurse is there to help you through this difficult time and offer both physical and emotional support as you become more confident.

> Remind yourself that you have had major surgery. Learn to celebrate every little achievement on the road to recovery.

Stoma care is just like any other skill you have had to learn, the more you practise and actively participate in your stoma care, the quicker you will become independent and stoma care will become part of your daily routine.

Day 1 post-surgery – the day after your surgery will be very busy for you. You will be expected to start mobilising around the ward and be out of bed for at least 6 hours, eat and drink. Your PCA or epidural pain relief may be switched to tablet form. Your stoma nurse will come to teach you how to change your bag and care for your stoma and you will be encouraged to participate.

Day 2 post-surgery – you will be expected to mobilise around the ward and be out of bed for at least 8 hours. It is preferable if you put on your normal clothes rather than walking around in a hospital gown, as this will make you feel much better. You will be eating and drinking as tolerated. You will need to change your stoma bag under supervision of your stoma nurse or the ward nurse. While it is normal to feel unsure and seek assistance from your nurse, it will help you gain confidence with your stoma care if you try to do as much as possible independently. It is advisable that you use the time in hospital to practise. If you feel up to it, you may be supervised twice a day to become proficient. You may even be able to cut your baseplate or practise emptying your stoma bag without the direct supervision of your stoma nurse. When emptying your stoma bag make sure that you or ward staff records your output, as it is important to know how much output is being produced from your stoma.

Day 3–4 post-surgery – depending on your progress, you may be ready to go home on day 3 or 4 post-surgery. In order to be fit for discharge, your surgeon will make sure that all your tests are within normal range, you are feeling well, eating and drinking, mobilising independently and your stoma is working. Most importantly, your stoma nurse will need to review you and make sure that you are independent with your stoma care. If you cannot care for your stoma yourself, we may need to teach a member of your family who will be able to care for your stoma. Stoma nurses in the community cannot come to your house daily to care for your stoma so you or a family member must be able to care for your stoma before discharge. If your GP considers that it will be appropriate for you to have a package of care or if you have your own private carers, the stoma nurse will ensure they know how to care for your stoma before you are discharged from the hospital.

Day of discharge – once everyone has agreed that you can go home, you will receive your hospital discharge letter and if required, medications to take home. An outpatient appointment to see your surgeon will be sent in the post separately. **Local residents with a GP in Harrow, Brent or Ealing, will be given an outpatient appointment with the stoma nurses from St Mark's Hospital** in approximately 2 weeks post-surgery and also provided with telephone support for up to ten days immediately following discharge home. If you are unable to attend clinic we will offer you a home visit though these are reserved for patients that are unable to travel easily or require extra support.

Discharge home checklist

- [ ] 1–2 weeks of stoma supplies
- [ ] St Mark's Hospital stoma nurse contact details
- [ ] Stoma clinic appointment for follow-up or your local stoma nurses' details
- [ ] Telephone home support service contact details (if local)
- [ ] Copy of stoma care discharge letter and prescription request for your records
- [ ] Dispensing Appliance Contractor (DAC) or Prescription Management Service contact numbers

If you have been referred from a GP or hospital outside our catchment area, you will be referred to a stoma nurse at your local hospital. **Contact your local stoma nurse in the first instance** rather than the St Mark's Hospital stoma nurses as they are able to help you with any issues, visit you at home if necessary or see you in their outpatient clinic. **Appendix 1 details the St Mark's Hospital stoma patient pathway.**

Stoma supplies and prescription management at home

Your stoma nurse will give you enough stoma supplies to last for 1–2 weeks, as well as discussing your options to receive stoma supplies at home. A prescription needs to be raised by your GP or stoma nurse before the stoma supplies are dispensed or delivered.

If you live in England, you may need to pay for your prescription. You are entitled to prescription charge exemption if you have a permanent stoma, are over 60 years old, if you have cancer or if you already were exempt from prescription charges for other reasons. If you have a temporary stoma, you will have to pay for prescriptions, unless you have cancer. Your GP can help you apply for a prescription exemption certificate. If you are going to need three or more prescriptions within three months or 13 or more prescriptions in 12 months, then you should consider applying for a prescription prepayment certificate (PPC), which will reduce the cost for all prescriptions, including stoma care products and medications. You can discuss with your GP any issues relevant to PPC or prescription exemption certificates.

> You are at liberty to change the method of how you receive your products at any time but you will need to discuss this with your GP or prescribing hub so your prescription is sent to the correct dispenser.

Once home you will be issued with a prescription for all your stoma products to last for **one month, receive complementary dry wipes and rubbish bags with every order** and be offered **free delivery** to your home or an address of your choice, regardless of which option you choose.

There are three options for obtaining your stoma products and it is completely up to you to decide which option suits you best.

Option 1: Dispensing appliance contractor (DAC)

Your stoma nurse will register you with a DAC (stoma products delivery company) and arrange for them to deliver your products. Your order usually takes around 1 week to arrive as you have to allow time for the GP to receive the prescription request from the stoma nurse and write a prescription. You can choose if you want to collect your prescription from the GP or let the DAC collect the prescription on your behalf. Once the DAC receives the prescription they need to process it, dispense the products and arrange a mutually convenient time for delivery. The DAC will contact you about 2 weeks before you need to reorder to remind you and to check if your products are still suitable. DACs offer an appliance cutting service for patients that are unable to cut their stoma appliance but this should be requested through the stoma nurse.

Option 2: Nurse-led prescribing hubs

If this option is available in your area, your stoma nurse will send your prescription request directly to the hub and you should receive your supplies within a few days. The prescribing hub will process, dispense and deliver all your stoma products without having to involve your GP as the prescription is managed by experienced stoma nurses who can prescribe your products. The hub will contact you about 2 weeks before you need to reorder to remind you and to check if your products are still suitable. A prescribing hub can offer an appliance cutting service for patients that are unable to cut their stoma appliance and this is requested through the stoma nurse.

Option 3: Collect from a local pharmacy

Your stoma nurse will send your discharge letter with your **initial** prescription request to your GP. If you choose to collect your stoma products from your local pharmacy, you will need to either collect your **repeat** prescriptions from your GP first and give it to your pharmacy or ask your GP to send the prescription to your chosen pharmacy. The prescription request may take a few days to get to your GP and then another few days for the prescription to be sent to the pharmacy of your choice. Unlike a DAC or prescribing hub who hold stoma stock in multiple warehouses, your pharmacy may not have all the stoma supplies you need at their premises and you may need to wait slightly longer for them to be delivered or you may receive a part order. When you have about two weeks of stoma supplies left, you will need to contact your GP and request a repeat prescription, which will then need to get to your pharmacy. If you have requested that your bags are cut to a particular size before you collect them, you may also have to wait slightly longer as the pharmacy usually has to arrange for an appliance cutting service off site, unlike a DAC or prescribing hub who has on-site cutting facilities.

 If you receive stock you no longer need or receive more than you use, inform your GP, prescribing hub or DAC so they update your prescription. Stoma products that are issued but unused cannot be returned and this is at great cost to the NHS.

Sampling of stoma products

Ideally before hospital discharge, you would have a discussion with your stoma nurse about different stoma appliances that are available on prescription. You may already know which stoma bag you want to use as this may have been discussed when you visited your stoma nurse before your operation or you may have done your own research or sampled a variety of bags. However, as your time in hospital is usually very limited and focused on you learning how to look after your stoma and recover from surgery, most patients feel too overwhelmed to sample different products and are happy to be discharged on the stoma appliance they were trained with. Once you become more confident with your stoma care you may find it beneficial to sample other stoma appliances, especially if you feel that the brand you are using is no longer suitable for your current requirements or lifestyle. Sampling other products is not essential if you are confident with your products and your stoma care. You can obtain samples by:

- contacting stoma appliance manufacturers via telephone or online
- contacting national support groups or stoma associations
- contacting your DAC or prescribing hub
- contacting your stoma nurse
- visiting patient open days
- joining local or national support groups and receiving samples or product updates with their magazines
- speaking to other people with a stoma

> 🦁 If you need to add, substitute or try new products, you must contact your stoma nurse to ensure the products are suitable for you before they can be added to your prescription.

Nurse-led stoma care outpatient clinics

Stoma care clinics are for new and established stoma patients to attend for routine check-ups, complication management, emotional support and general lifestyle advice. Most stoma care clinics are not available on weekends, bank holidays or after 6pm on weekdays and therefore are not emergency services. The clinics are by **appointments only** and the venue depends on where you are registered with your GP. You can make an appointment by contacting the stoma care department directly or by getting a referral from your GP, if you have not seen a stoma nurse for some time or recently moved into the area.

Your stoma nurse will continue to see you in an outpatient clinic for as long as you need to be seen but this could be either in a face-to-face, telephone or virtual clinic (using your smartphone or computer). If you have a non-urgent question, we also provide an email service. Telephone messages and emails may not be answered immediately as stoma nurses may be with other patients but you can always leave a message and a stoma nurse will get back to you as soon as possible. **Always remember to leave your full name, contact details and hospital number, NHS number or date of birth** so we can answer your query. It is advisable to contact us sooner rather than later if you are concerned about your stoma to prevent the problem getting worse.

Ideally you should be reviewed **annually** by your stoma nurse to ensure you are using the most suitable products for your stoma and to have an opportunity to discuss any concerns you may have. Sometimes we may invite you to provide feedback on your visit or assist us with research or audits to improve the service we offer, however, this is not compulsory.

 If you need to see a stoma nurse or have any other concerns with your health outside our working hours, contact the out of hours services.

2. General stoma care

The first few steps of adjusting to life with a stoma is learning how to care for your stoma, become confident managing your stoma on a daily basis and regain an acceptable quality of life. It will take practice to develop techniques that work well for your lifestyle and gain a better understanding of the different stoma products available on the market. There are various accessory products to assist with stoma care but you should always start with as few items as possible and only use additional accessories if needed or advised by your stoma nurse.

Basic stoma care – step-by-step bag change

Before attempting to change your stoma bag, get everything ready:

- adhesive remover spray
- rubbish bag
- a bowl of warm tap water
- dry wipes or non-sterile gauze swabs
- stoma measuring guide or pre-cut template
- a pair of scissors
- a pen or marker
- new stoma bag

Optional: mirror and paper towels

1. **Empty your bag** – if it is drainable. Colostomy bags are closed and therefore emptying is not required.

2. **Remove used bag** – using a remover spray gently pull the used bag off your skin. Lift the tab to ensure the spray goes **between** your skin and the bag. Hold your skin with one finger when separating the bag from your skin to prevent tearing your skin. Place the used stoma bag into your rubbish bag.

3. **Clean the stoma and surrounding skin** – wet a few wipes or gauze swabs to remove any residual stoma output. Use dry wipes or gauze swabs to dry the skin properly.

4. **Measure the stoma** – using the measuring guide. Not all stoma shapes are round, therefore, you may need to measure it top to bottom (height) and side to side (width) to make an accurate template. A mirror may be helpful to ensure the measurement is correct.

5. **Cut the baseplate** – once you have measured the size of your stoma, use

a pen to draw the shape on your baseplate. Then use a pair of scissors to cut the appropriate shape. A pre-cut baseplate will not need cutting.

6. **Remove the protective backing** – from your baseplate. The plastic backing can be dated and kept as a reference template.

7. **Position the bag** – over the stoma and stick onto your skin. Press the baseplate around the stoma and surrounding skin to ensure good adherence. Ensure that the bottom of your bag is closed, if you are using a drainable appliance. Dispose of used stoma bag and wipes in your normal household waste bin.

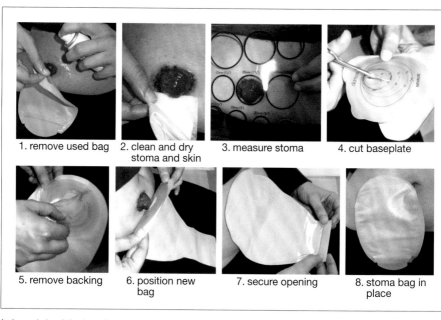

1. remove used bag   2. clean and dry stoma and skin   3. measure stoma   4. cut baseplate

5. remove backing   6. position new bag   7. secure opening   8. stoma bag in place

It is advisable to change your stoma bag before you eat or drink or wait a couple of hours after a meal as your stoma will be less active. You may notice that there is a certain time of the day that your stoma is less active and this may be an ideal opportunity to change your stoma bag. If you are concerned with the possible unpleasant odour while changing your stoma bag, follow the tips below:

- ensure good ventilation in the room you are changing your stoma bag
- use scented candles, oil burner, room freshener or an aroma diffuser
- use a neutralising air freshener which can be purchased from a supermarket
- when changing your stoma bag add 1–2 drops of lavender or mint essential oil into the bag to help neutralise odour which can be purchased from a supermarket.

Types of stoma bags

There are many different brands, designs and sizes of stoma bags and it may be overwhelming to know which one is right for you. Some people continue to use the bag they have become accustomed to in hospital while others try a variety of bags before settling on a certain product.

Your stoma nurse will be at hand to help you choose the correct bag or to assist you if you need advice or develop problems with your stoma bag.

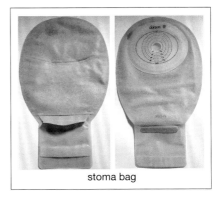
stoma bag

If for any reason you would like to change your stoma bag, you must seek the advice of your stoma nurse first to ensure that the bag is appropriate for your stoma, as not every bag on the market will be suitable for your specific needs.

How to choose the ideal stoma bag?

A combination of factors determines which stoma bag is best for you and depends on the type of stoma formed, daily volume of output produced, where the stoma is positioned on your abdomen and your individual lifestyle choices.

Not all manufacturing companies produce the full range of products but your stoma nurse will be able to help you choose the stoma appliance that best fits your needs.

If you are unable to cut your own baseplates, your stoma nurse can request to have these delivered pre-cut.

1. Opening – first determine which stoma bag is best for you by deciding if you need **a foldable opening, a tap or no opening**. This will depend on which stoma you have or the output.

Foldable opening – this type of stoma bag is drainable and has a foldable opening at the bottom, allowing you to empty the content without having to change the stoma bag each time it becomes full. You can roll the bag up and close it with the help of a Velcro strip or a clip that secures the opening of the bag. It is usually used for a stoma with loose output, requiring multiple emptying throughout the day, such as an ileostomy. However, drainable bags can also be used for a colostomy when the output is loose.

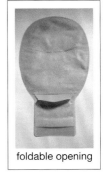
foldable opening

Tap opening – this type of stoma bag has a tap-like opening to empty the content and is found on high output and urostomy bags.

- **High output bag** – has a **tap opening** and larger capacity, which allows for better management of high output stomas such as high output ileostomy and jejunostomy. The tap also allows for a night drainage bag to be connected to the high output stoma bag and avoids frequent trips to the bathroom during the night. They may also be used in the immediate post-operative period if the output of the stoma is very liquid and/or high volume. It is advisable to switch to a bag with a foldable opening once the output thickens as it would become difficult to empty the contents through a tap opening.

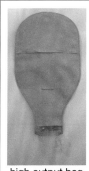
high output bag

- **Urostomy bag** – is a drainable bag **with a tap** that allows you to empty urine. It also has an anti-reflux valve, preventing your urine from flowing back to the urostomy, which prevents possible infection. You will need to empty your urostomy bag a few times throughout the day. You may also need to connect your urostomy bag to a night drainage bag to avoid having to wake up to empty your bag.

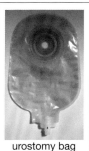
urostomy bag

No opening – this type of stoma bag is known as a **closed bag** since it does not have an opening at the bottom, hence you will need to change the entire bag each time it becomes full. It is only used for a colostomy, as the output is usually more formed and does not require multiple emptying throughout the day.

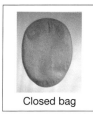
Closed bag

2. Baseplate – secondly you need to choose the most appropriate baseplate. A baseplate, also known as a flange or wafer, is the sticky part of your stoma bag which keeps the bag in place and protects your skin from the stoma output. Your stoma baseplate could either be **flat, convex or concave**.

flat baseplate

Flat baseplate – this type of baseplate is usually used for stomas with regular surrounding skin, without any skin creases, dips or folds. A flat baseplate is usually the first choice to start with.

convex baseplate

Convex baseplate – this type of baseplate is bulkier in comparison to a flat one. It is usually used when the skin surrounding the stoma has dips, creases and folds in order to allow a better adherence. A convex baseplate may also be useful if your stoma is not raised above the skin and you are experiencing leakages, as it helps raise the stoma above the skin level by pushing the surrounding skin downwards.

> ⚠ Only use a convex baseplate if advised by your stoma nurse as convexity can cause peristomal skin complications if not used properly.

Concave baseplate – this type of baseplate curves inwards like the inside of a bowl. It is usually used when the area around your stoma is curved, bulging or if you have a hernia around the stoma. This type of baseplate is more flexible and wraps around a bulge to keep your stoma bag in place.

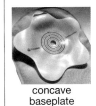

concave baseplate

3. System – you can then choose if you would prefer a **one-piece system or two-piece system**. This is usually a personal choice, however, some manufacturers may only produce a certain appliance in either a one or two-piece system.

One-piece – this type of system has the baseplate and the bag attached together as one piece. During bag changing, both the bag and the baseplate are removed.

Two-piece – this type of system has a separate baseplate and bag. This allows you to change your baseplate less often, every 2–3 days but change your bag more often. A two-piece

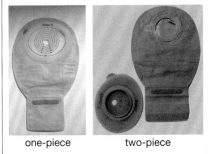

one-piece   two-piece

system may be useful if you have a colostomy that requires 1–3 bag changes a day, if you have a closed bag and need to let the air out, or when you need to perform regular procedures on the stoma but do not want to change your bag each time.

4. Capacity – there are different sizes of stoma bags – **mini, midi and maxi** which hold on average 250 ml, 420 ml and 550 ml respectively. Though smaller bags may be more discreet, the smaller your stoma bag is the more frequently you would need to empty it, therefore, most people wear a midi sized bag.

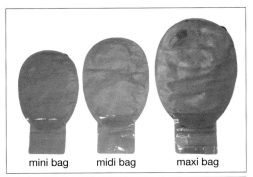

mini bag   midi bag   maxi bag

Stoma cap – is a tiny stoma appliance/bag that is usually applied over your stoma or mucous fistula when there is not much output. You can also wear a stoma cap if you irrigate your stoma.

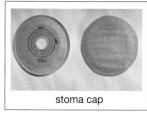

stoma cap

5. Appearance – your stoma bag can be **clear, opaque with a viewing option or completely opaque**. Depending on your lifestyle preferences you may choose the one that suits you best.

Clear – is a transparent bag that allows for your stoma and output to be visible and therefore more easily monitored. It is usually used immediately after surgery in order for nursing and medical staff to be able to see the stoma colour and monitor the output. However, some people choose to continue using a clear stoma bag on discharge from hospital.

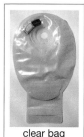

clear bag

Opaque with viewing option – is an opaque bag with a small flap in the middle of the bag that may be lifted to allow for your stoma and the output to be seen and easily monitored without being fully transparent.

Opaque – is a bag that hides the stoma and output completely. You will not be able to view the stoma or its contents without removing or emptying the bag.

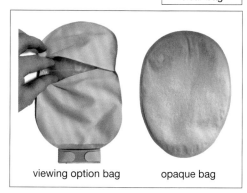

viewing option bag   opaque bag

Accessory stoma products

Sometimes you may develop complications with the stoma or surrounding skin and may need additional accessory products to resolve the issue. Ideally you should seek advice from your stoma nurse to help you navigate the extensive range available and teach you how to use these products effectively, as inappropriate use may not resolve your problem and could even make matters worse.

Adhesive remover spray/wipes – are used to remove a used stoma bag from your skin. Alternatively, if you are unable to use the spray you can use one adhesive remover wipe every time you need to change your bag. Wipes are handy for travelling or putting in hand luggage.

Stoma paste – is used to fill skin dips and deep creases which may otherwise cause your bag to leak.

Stoma rings/seals/washers – are used to fill skin dips and creases and can be likened to 'donuts'. Stoma rings are also used to treat skin damage or protect the skin if the stoma is at skin level or the stoma output is high and of liquid consistency. Stoma rings are soft and mouldable and can be cut to better fit around the stoma or rolled to fill deeper dips and creases.

Stoma powder – is used to help heal excoriated skin (broken/wet skin) and should be used sparingly until healing has occurred and then be discontinued.

Barrier wipes/spray – is usually used to create an extra barrier between the skin and stoma output in select patients. They should not be used for general skin protection or as a cleansing product.

Flange extenders – also known as security frames or elastic tape, but can be likened to 'bananas', 'half-moons' or 'smileys'. They can be attached to the outer edge of your baseplate and your skin providing additional support and security. They are used to help keep your stoma bag in place if you are experiencing a frequent or premature detachment of your stoma bag usually caused by a parastomal hernia or skin dip or if you wear your appliance for an extended period of time.

> ⚠ Flange extenders should not be used to 'patch' a leaking bag, as untreated leakage underneath the baseplate will cause excoriation to your skin.

Belt for convex bag – these belts are designed to provide extra security and keep your stoma bag in place. They can be attached to the belt loops located on each side of a convex stoma bag. They are usually used when your stoma is not well spouted and it is at the level of your skin. The belt would create extra pressure to the surrounding skin and help the stoma raise above the skin level.

Stoma shield/protector – looks like a small plastic shield, meant to provide extra protection for your stoma, especially when playing contact sports, playing with small children or large animals and if you work in an area where someone may accidentally bump into your stoma. It comes in different colours, shapes and sizes and you may benefit from speaking to your stoma nurse for fitting.

Thickener tablets/sachets – contain solidifying agents that help thicken your stoma output. You should not use them routinely as they can mask stoma problems such as loose and high output. It is advisable to use them only after consulting your stoma nurse. Most people use them when going out as they thicken their stoma output and reduce the risk of accidental leakages.

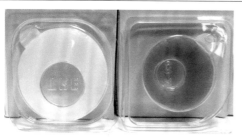
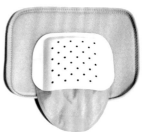

stoma rings   stoma shield / protector

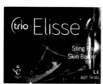
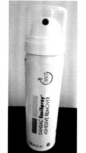
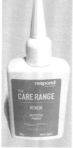
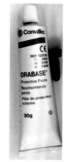
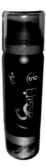

adhesive remover wipes, barrier wipes, adhesive remover spray,
stoma powder, Orabase paste, barrier spray

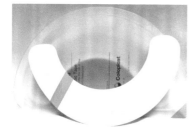

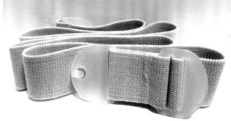

flange extenders   belt for convex bag

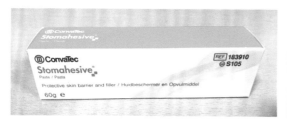
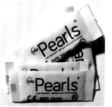

stoma paste   thickener sachets

Diet with a stoma

These recommendations serve only as a guide and must be personalised to **individual need and stoma type**. Dietary needs vary as do personal eating habits and lifestyle, therefore, if you require specialised nutritional advice, you should speak with your GP or ask to be referred to a dietitian.

Immediately after formation of a stoma, the intestine initially moves slower, due to the effect of the anaesthetic drugs used in the operation. Also a portion of your intestine will no longer be participating in the digestive process, therefore, the remaining intestine will need to adapt over time and adjust to absorbing more nutrients, water and salts. This adjustment period usually takes up to 6 weeks but mainly **depends on the type of stoma** you have and how much functioning intestine remains above your stoma. Some people may need a bit longer before their intestine fully adapts to its new role. While your intestine is adapting to its new role, you may have quite a liquid stoma output, so it is advisable to allow 20–30 minutes between eating and drinking to give your intestine time to digest the food.

Your intestine will initially be swollen from being handled in the operation and needs time to recover. During this recovery time, your intestinal function is quite erratic and food may pass through quickly and cause a more liquid and high output. **Avoiding irritant foods like high fibre, spicy and high-fat/ processed foods** will allow your intestine to settle down and also prevent intestinal obstruction, excessive wind or crampy abdominal pain. Spicy foods may irritate your intestine and increase your stoma output but if you are used to a spicy diet you may find you can tolerate spices much earlier after surgery but you should still be cautious. It is important to follow a certain diet in order to prevent dehydration and electrolyte deficits, which is more common with a stoma in the small intestine. **Salt** is an important mineral that may be lost in your stoma output and must be replaced either by sprinkling approximately a teaspoon a day of table salt over your food or drinking fluids which are high in salt.

A poor appetite after your surgery is normal but you need to stimulate the intestine to work by eating small meals more frequently and also adding snacks, as it is likely you will not tolerate three large meals throughout the day. Carbohydrate and protein rich foods are usually easier to digest, so are good first choices when you are allowed to eat again. It is important to **eat nutrient rich foods from all three categories: carbohydrates, proteins and fats** to help your body heal and prevent infection.

Immediately post-operation (fluids only)

You will need to follow a standard post-surgery diet to prevent complications and restore intestinal function.

Clear fluids

Immediately after you wake up from your surgery, you will be allowed to have some sips of water. If you tolerate sips of water, without feeling nauseated or vomiting, you will be able to progress to having clear fluids such as:

Clear fluids		
Coffee (no milk)	Clear soup	Fruit juice (no pulp)
Tea (no milk)	Bouillon	Water
Jelly	Non-fat stock	Squash
Ice pops (no milk)		

Free fluids

Once you are able to tolerate clear fluids, you may progress your diet to free fluids, which can include any type of fluids, without any restrictions.

Free fluids		
Milk	Fruit juices with pulp	Coffee with milk
Soups	Ice cream	Milkshakes
Soy/almond/rice drinks	Tea with milk	Supplement drinks
Yogurt	Custard	

New stoma diet (up to 6 weeks)

Once you are able to tolerate fluids, you will progress to eating solids, starting with a low fibre diet and building up to a normal diet as possible. This transition may take up to 6 weeks or longer depending on how well you recover.

A low fibre diet includes foods that are easy to digest, reducing the risk of increased stoma output, obstruction, wind, bloating and abdominal pain. Insoluble fibre is avoided on a low fibre diet but allows soluble fibre as tolerated. It is important to be able to understand the different types of fibre and monitor the effect they have on your stoma output.

- **Insoluble fibre** – usually found in seeds, whole grains, bran, nuts, corn, brown rice, fruit peels, etc. It cannot be dissolved in water and your intestine does not break it down. Insoluble fibre **adds bulk to the stool and helps food pass more quickly**, which may increase your stoma output.

- **Soluble fibre** – usually found in porridge, bananas, apples, carrots, barley, etc. It dissolves in water and forms gel-like material. It draws water to your gut, which helps your stool become soft. **This slows digestion process and would help slow your stoma output.**

Avoid high-fat/processed foods – while it is important to eat high calorie and high-protein foods to help with your recovery, it is best if you avoid food high in fat and some processed foods, as these may increase your stoma output.

Foods that are prepared by roasting/ baking or boiling are easier to digest and are healthier choices. If your appetite is very poor and you have lost weight prior to your surgery, it is better to choose foods that are higher in fats, though this does not necessarily mean choosing unhealthy foods.

You can replace low-fat yogurt or milk with full-fat options, add butter to your mashed potatoes or bread, add olive oil or grated cheese to your pasta and double cream to soup.

This should help you regain your weight and build up your energy. Small portions of cakes, crisps and biscuits as a snack, are encouraged. **Appendix 2 details examples of meal plans for a new stoma diet.**

Foods to include

White pasta/bread/rice	Fish, lean meats, poultry
Crackers without nuts and seeds	Milk, cheese, yogurt
Biscuits without nuts and seeds	Eggs
Peeled potatoes	Apple sauce
Refined cereals (Rice Krispies, Corn Flakes)	Bananas (ripe)
	Peeled tinned fruit and vegetables
Porridge	Peeled cooked fruit and vegetables
Smooth peanut butter	Fruit/vegetable juice without pulp
Soy/almond/rice drinks	Clear jelly, ice cream (no nuts/fruit)
Mashed/pureed vegetables without skin	Soups (cream soups, broth, stock)
	Tofu
Rice pudding, tapioca, custard	

Foods to avoid

Wholemeal pasta	Fruit and vegetables with seeds
Brown or wild rice	Fruit/vegetable juice with pulp
Wholegrain/wholemeal bread	Prunes and prune juice
Bread with nuts/fruit	Mushrooms
Wholegrain cereals (bran, Weetabix®)	Corn and popcorn
	Spicy foods
Cereals with nuts	Fruit preserves with seeds
Nuts and seeds	Marmalade
Dried fruit, tinned pineapples	Tough/gristle-rich meat
Unpeeled potatoes	Coconut
Berries	Dried beans, peas, lentils, chickpeas
Cabbage, sauerkraut, broccoli, cauliflower with stalk	Crunchy peanut butter
Raw unpeeled fruit/vegetable	Wholegrain chapatti bread
Leafy greens	

Irritant drinks/fluids – certain drinks may also have a direct effect on your intestine causing increased stoma output, wind or even contribute to severe dehydration. It is, therefore, important to include certain fluids and avoid others in the first few weeks following surgery.

Drinks to include
Decaffeinated coffee/tea or herbal tea (except green and black tea)
Water, coconut water or squash
Milk or kefir
Meat/vegetable stock, soup (strained), savoury drinks (Bovril®, Oxo®, Knorr®)
Non-fizzy sports drinks (Lucozade®, Powerade®, Gatorade®)
Foods rich in water (melon, yogurt)

Drinks to avoid
Alcohol
Caffeinated drinks (tea, coffee, energy drinks, coke)
High sugar/artificial sugar content drinks (too much fruit juice, some energy and sports drinks)
Fizzy drinks

Established stoma diet (after 4–6 weeks)

Having a stoma does not necessarily mean that you will not be able to enjoy the foods or drinks you used to enjoy before your surgery. The aim is to gradually return to your normal diet and if that cannot be completely achieved, a diet with minimal limitations. With instruction from your surgeon and stoma nurse, you can now start to gradually introduce the foods from the 'avoid lists' mentioned above. If a particular food causes you problems, such as increased stoma output, bloating, excessive wind or cramps, stop eating it and avoid it for a few more weeks.

Tips to remember when reintroducing foods:

- try new foods one at a time
- reintroduce foods in small quantities
- take note of the effect of certain foods that you think may be an irritant
- try each new food at least **three** times before you completely eliminate it from your diet and give yourself a few weeks between each trial

- chew your food well as digestion starts in your mouth
- contact your stoma nurse if you are concerned about the stoma output, consistency or volume

 If you progress to a specific diet stage but experience abdominal discomfort, cramps and/or bloating, go back a stage and then try progressing again as tolerated.

Foods and their effect on stoma output – the following food charts are to help you in making food choices but remember that certain foods will have a different effect on different people and will also depend on your specific stoma type. Be mindful of the effect of certain foods and drinks on your stoma output and eat them as tolerated.

May increase stoma output			
Alcohol Coffee, tea Fruit juices, prune/apple juice Spicy foods	Fried foods Prunes Whole grains Raisins Brown bread Brown rice	Milk Raw vegetables Leafy greens Chocolate Baked beans	Broccoli, cauliflower, cabbage Fresh fruits Brown pasta Wholemeal chapatti bread

May thicken stoma output		
Marshmallows Jelly babies Bananas Mashed potatoes	White bread/toast/pasta Peeled potatoes Tapioca pudding	Boiled white rice Apple sauce Yogurt Smooth peanut butter

May cause stoma obstruction		
Nuts, seeds Mushrooms Sweetcorn Popcorn Fruit/vegetable skins Dried fruit	Pineapples, oranges Coleslaw Raw fruit/vegetables Pith (white stringy bits) Coconut Peas	Chinese vegetables Shrimp, lobster Celery Leafy greens Vegetable stalks

May increase stoma odour			
Asparagus	Garlic	Peanut butter	Sprouts
Fish	Strong cheese	Cabbage	Broccoli
Onion	Eggs	Cauliflower	Baked beans

May reduce stoma odour		
Tomato juice	Buttermilk	Peppermint water
Orange juice	Cranberry juice	Peppermint tea
Yogurt	Parsley	Peppermint capsules

May change colour of stoma output	
Red (tomato juice, red wine, beetroot, red berries, blackcurrant drinks)	Black (iron, charcoal, liquorice)
	Antibiotics (grey, red, green)
Food colouring or dyes	Antacids (white, grey)

May cause increased wind (flatus)		
Broccoli, cauliflower, cabbage, sprouts	Eggs	Alcohol
Mushrooms	Bran	Cucumber
Fried/fatty foods	Onions, garlic	Chewing gum
Fruit skins	Nuts, seeds	Sweetcorn
Creamy foods, dairy products, cheese	Dried fruit	Asparagus
Lentils, soy, beans, peas	Fizzy drinks	
Peanut butter		

Non dietary tips to reduce wind:

- chew your food well
- avoid chewing gum
- avoid talking while eating
- take your time and eat slowly
- eat regularly and do not skip meals
- avoid drinking through a straw
- limit high fibre foods

- avoid fizzy drinks or pour your drink in a glass, stir and allow to settle
- use wind reducing tablets which contain charcoal, peppermint or Simethicone

Special diets

If you had any underlying medical conditions or special diets prior to your stoma surgery, you may need extra support to find a diet which does not compromise your ongoing medical treatment, special diet or stoma function. **Some dietary modifications will be necessary, especially in the first 6 weeks** after your stoma formation and you or your stoma nurse may need to consult your GP, dietician or specialist practitioner for advice.

Diabetics – you must continue to follow your recommended diabetic diet, but some modifications may be required. The following tips should help you better manage your diabetes and stoma:

- **Measure your blood glucose levels** more often after stoma formation as your food intake post-surgery would not be the same as it was before as you would most likely need to eat **foods that are high in calories and carbohydrates,** and this could lead to changes in your **blood glucose levels (blood sugar).**
- Keep a food chart to find out which foods work best and those to avoid or use sparingly.
- If you are on diabetic medications you may require a specialist review to adjust the dose of your insulin or tablets.
- Some people who usually manage their diabetes with diet alone may benefit from using diabetic medication until you find the right balance with your stoma.
- Some people who are on tablets need to swap to insulin until the correct balance is reached.
- Depending on how much intestine was removed, especially if you have a **small intestine stoma**, you may not be able to absorb the diabetic tablets you used to take before your operation, therefore, you will need to speak to your GP or diabetic specialist and discuss whether your medications need adjusting or switching to a different type.

- If your diabetic diet requires high fibre foods that may increase your stoma output, you may need medications that help reduce your stoma output such as Loperamide and Codeine Phosphate

Vegans and vegetarians – you can continue to follow a vegan/vegetarian diet long term but initially after surgery you must:

- Eat fruit and vegetables that are low in fibre and easy to digest such as mashed/pureed peeled vegetables and fruits, peeled cooked vegetables and fruits, ripe bananas, peeled potatoes, tinned fruit and vegetables without skin.

- Avoid fruit and vegetables that may increase your stoma output, increase wind and odour or cause an obstruction.

- As protein is important for wound healing some strict vegan and vegetarian diets may lack protein and it is advisable that you consider food substitutes such as tofu, soy, Quorn™.

- **Ileostomy or jejunostomy** patients are at a higher risk of vitamin B_{12} deficiency. Additionally being vegan or vegetarian may increase your likelihood of B_{12} deficiency as it is usually found in animal products. Therefore it is advisable that you eat vitamin B_{12} fortified foods such as cereals and bread or add supplements to your diet.

- Organise a blood test with your GP if you are worried about your weight or nutritional intake.

Coeliac disease – unfortunately your stoma does not cure coeliac disease but you may find your symptoms are better after your operation, however, you will need to continue to follow your special gluten-free diet.

Lactose intolerance – having a stoma does not change your pre-existing lactose intolerance condition and you should continue to avoid foods and drinks with lactose and replace them with lactose-free products. However, some patients with a mild lactose intolerance may find they can manage their bowel frequency better with a stoma than before their operation, so may continue to have small quantities of lactose-based food or drinks. Some patients may have simply avoided lactose products prior to surgery as it made their pre-existing condition worse and were therefore never diagnosed with a true lactose intolerance. These patients usually find lactose products more digestible following surgery if introduced slowly.

Kidney disease – if you have underlying kidney problems you may have been advised to avoid certain foods such as protein, salt and potassium rich foods and may even have to abide to a strict fluid restriction, therefore you should consult your specialist doctor and dietician and decide together the best diet for your new stoma. **It is more important you continue to follow your kidney disease management plan rather than the stoma diet** but you should be able to make certain adjustments to balance the two conditions.

- Consult your GP or specialist doctor or dietician if you are considering adding certain foods/drinks to your diet.

- Have your **kidney function bloods** and **urine sodium** checked more regularly by your GP, so that any abnormalities could be treated promptly before any serious complications occur. Abnormal kidney function bloods and urine sodium levels are a good indication of dehydration.

High blood pressure – if you have high blood pressure you probably have been advised to reduce or avoid salt. Having a **stoma in the small intestine** often requires increasing your salt intake as you lose salts in your stoma output. As salt plays an important role in managing your stoma and your blood pressure, you will need to learn to balance the two conditions.

- **Check your blood pressure** more often so that you can see how your new diet is affecting your blood pressure.
- Inform your GP or cardiologist of any abnormalities, as they may need to adjust your medications accordingly.
- While it is important to replace any salts lost through your stoma output, always consult your GP whether it is appropriate to add more salt to your diet.
- Adjust your diet and try healthier choices by avoiding high salt, processed and fried foods that may worsen your blood pressure.

Heart conditions – you may have been told by your GP or cardiologist to avoid drinking too much fluids but advised by your stoma nurse to drink approximately 1.5–2 litres of fluids a day. If you need to limit your fluid intake due to a heart condition:

- Consult your GP or cardiologist whether it is appropriate for you to add more salt rather than more fluids to your diet.
- Consult your GP or cardiologist and ask if it is appropriate for you to drink more fluids rich in salt such as St Mark's E–mix solution, vegetable/meat stock, Bovril®, Oxo®.
- Monitor very carefully how much you drink and how much you lose through your stoma in order to make sure that you are not losing too much fluid or that you are not drinking too much. For an accurate fluid balance, you can measure your stoma output by emptying your stoma bag into a plastic measuring jug, before discarding the contents into the toilet.
- However, if you only need an estimate output, it may be more convenient to fill a stoma bag with the amount of water you usually empty from your bag, and then pour the water in a measuring cup so you can see how much intestinal content approximately is lost each time you empty your bag.
- Remember or document how many times a day you empty your bag in a 24–hour period.
- You can use a small notepad and write down what you drink and what you lose from your stoma bag.

Food allergies – your stoma does not change your allergy status and you should continue to exclude all foods and/or medications as you used to do before your operation.

> If you are losing too much fluid through your stoma, **add** more salt to your diet rather than drinking more liquids but you must consult your GP or stoma nurse **first** if you have other medical conditions such as high blood pressure, kidney disease or heart conditions.

Medications with a stoma

Having a stoma may affect how you absorb certain medications particularly if you have had a large amount of intestine removed, experience episodes of vomiting or if you have a more liquid or high output stoma.

Therefore, medications that used to work well for you may no longer have the same effect after your surgery and you may need a different dose or form of medication.

If you find capsules, tablets or undigested tablets in your stoma bag, it **does not necessarily mean** that your medications are not being absorbed. Most **immediate release** and **uncoated** tablets and capsules can be crushed or opened to allow better absorption, however, always consult your pharmacist before crushing or opening tablets and capsules.

Modified release medications – such as slow release (prolonged release) medications are designed to release their content into your body slowly, reducing possible side effects and providing medication over a longer time, usually 12 or 24 hours. Sometimes they may be passed quickly into your stoma bag without giving them enough time to be absorbed and they may be ineffective.

Enteric-coated medications – have a coating that protects them from dissolving in the stomach as they are meant to be absorbed in your small intestine. Sometimes they may pass through your stoma before being fully absorbed or without being absorbed at all.

Liquid medications – if possible avoid liquid (elixir) mediations with high levels of alcohol, sugar or sugar-free medications containing Sorbitol and Xylitol, as these may increase stoma output.

> Never crush **modified release medications or enteric-coated medications** as crushing them may give you an overdose of medication or side effects, which may be dangerous to you.

Contraceptive pills – may not be absorbed adequately especially if you are vomiting or have a high output stoma, therefore, may not be as effective. Speak to your sexual health clinic to discuss other forms of contraception if you are concerned about getting pregnant.

Antibiotics – may disrupt your gut flora and cause a more liquid stool and/or high output from your stoma, however, in some cases your stoma output may thicken. Either way, you should not alter your dose and should finish your course as prescribed.

Opioids – are a group of medications usually used for post-operative pain relief as they work well on severe pain but are also useful for long-term pain relief. These drugs can make you sleepy or relaxed and may even give you a feeling of pleasure in higher doses, therefore are usually advised to take at night, if possible. Opioids, such as Morphine or Codeine based medication are only available on prescription as they may also decrease your breathing and heart rate and can become addictive in high doses and if not monitored carefully. The common side effects of opioid medications are nausea, vomiting and constipation which can affect your stoma output. Sometimes opioid medication may be prescribed to thicken your stoma output.

Diuretic medication – or 'water pills' used to treat high blood pressure, heart failure, fluid overload or other conditions, may put you at risk of dehydration and electrolyte losses. While it is important to treat your other medical conditions, remind your doctor that you have a stoma especially if you are also asked to restrict your fluid intake. Some diuretics may cause greater loss of electrolytes such as potassium and it may be beneficial to use potassium sparing diuretics.

Metformin – is a medication that helps manage diabetes and generally does not cause problems with a stoma, but some people may experience more liquid or higher volume output when taking Metformin. If that is the case with you, it may be best to consult your GP or pharmacist and discuss different options.

Laxatives – may be suggested as part of bowel preparation for some investigations but can cause severe fluid and electrolytes losses and dehydration.

Digoxin – when you lose too much salt and potassium, your body may be unable to absorb Digoxin properly, causing an excessive amount of the medication to build up in your body, and this may cause toxicity and be quite harmful and dangerous for you. Potassium supplements may be advisable when taking Digoxin. Your GP should take regular blood tests to monitor your Digoxin and electrolytes levels. In addition, you should monitor for the following signs and symptoms of Digoxin toxicity:

- irregular pulse, fast or slow heartbeat

- loss of appetite, nausea, vomiting, diarrhoea
- confusion
- blurred vision

Warfarin – is a medication commonly used to thin the blood. You should **not** drink cranberry, grapefruit or pomegranate juice if you are on Warfarin, as it increases the effect of Warfarin and your blood may become too thin, while leafy greens may decrease the effect of Warfarin.

 Do not change your dose or stop taking your medication even if it affects your stoma output without **first** speaking to your GP, pharmacist or surgeon. They will be able to prescribe the right medication for your specific type of stoma.

Herbal remedies or food supplements – some people use alternative medication such as herbal medication or food supplements to enhance their physical or mental health. You must let your stoma nurse or GP know if you are taking alternative medication as sometimes these treatments may change your stoma output or interact with prescribed medication required for your stoma.

Ghost tablets phenomenon – sometimes you may pass what appears to be undigested tablets or capsules in your stoma bag. Usually this is just the shell or protective covering which holds the drug, as the actual active ingredient of the medication has already been absorbed in your body. This phenomenon is known as **'ghost pills'** or **'ghost tablets'** and is common with many modified release medications. However, in people with a high output ileostomy or jejunostomy, the medication may not actually be absorbed. If you feel you are not getting the benefits of your medication you must discuss this with your GP, as you may need a different form of medication.

 Always inform your GP or doctors that you have a stoma, as this should be taken into consideration when you are prescribed new medication or when you need a new treatment.

Adjusting to life with a stoma – hints and tips

The first few days after being discharged from hospital may be challenging for you. Arriving home and having to look after your stoma on your own, without the help of your stoma nurse may make you feel overwhelmed. Your stoma may be erratic, as you are readjusting to your daily routine and diet. You may experience stoma bag leaks or accidents but within a few days you will get into your own routine and your confidence will improve so that you can begin to resolve problems on your own. You will start to understand how your stoma functions, when it is more active and when it is less active and be able to adjust your diet or lifestyle accordingly. If you are struggling to cope, you can always contact your stoma nurse or you may find it more useful to speak to someone who has lived experience of life with a stoma, through making contact with a member of a support group. You can find a list of support groups in the **'psychological support'** section at the end of this book.

Storage – your stoma products can be bulky or difficult to store, so some people find it useful to buy a wheeled, plastic drawer tower storage unit. Use the different drawers to store your products by type as this will allow for quick access.

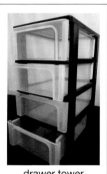

drawer tower storage

Emptying your bag – if your bag is drainable and you need to empty it into the toilet, it is advisable that you sit on the toilet and let your stoma bag drain in between your legs. You can sit as you normally would on the toilet or sit **facing the back** of the toilet, if easier. Some people choose to empty their stoma bag while standing, however, this may cause splashing and soiling.

It may be a good idea to put some toilet tissue inside the toilet bowl before emptying to reduce splashing. You could also face the toilet and bend onto your knees but this is not advisable in public toilets or if you have difficulty bending. Some people may empty the contents of the stoma bag into a bowl and then empty the bowl into the toilet. The bowl can be washed when the toilet is flushed and stored in the toilet for future use. Try to empty your bag when it is half full or after a meal to avoid overfilling.

Keep the opening clean – after emptying your stoma bag make sure you lift the opening/tap upwards to prevent the output leaking whilst you try to clean the bottom of the bag. You do not have to clean inside the opening/tap but care must be taken to dry the opening/tap properly as residual stoma output may cause an offensive odour or stain your underwear. A packet of wet wipes can be handy to clean the opening/tap of the stoma bag before closing it and also for wiping any residue which may come in contact with your hands to prevent staining on your bag.

Changing time – after surgery, your stoma may be erratic and unpredictable, but will settle into a routine and you should be able to find the best time of the day for changing your appliance. Many people with a stoma prefer to do so in the morning before breakfast but others change it later in the day, after a shower or before bed. What works for one person may not be the best choice for another, therefore, you should choose what works best for you and change your stoma bag accordingly.

Meal time – avoid changing your stoma bag immediately after eating or drinking as your stoma will be more active and it may be difficult to perform stoma care. Try changing your stoma bag **before** meals or 1–2 hours after a meal.

Going to bed – it is advisable to check/empty your bag before bed.

Extra wipes – if you run out of wipes or rubbish bags, you can contact your delivery company or pharmacy and request extra, free of charge. However, it is an idea to invest in some good quality paper towel (kitchen roll) which can be useful in mopping up stoma output or drying the area around the stoma, therefore saving your wipes for cleaning the stoma and surrounding skin.

Disposal of used bags – used stoma bags should be discarded in your normal household waste bin. However, if you find it difficult to do so, you can buy a nappy bin and use it for your stoma bags in the same way you would dispose of used baby nappies.

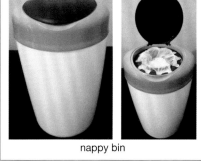

nappy bin

Going out – if you feel ready to go out, you may find it helpful and less stressful if you are prepared.

- Check, empty or change your bag (if closed) **before** going out and take spare stoma products with you.

- Wear comfortable clothes that you can easily access your stoma bag if you need to.

- Check the stoma bag regularly to prevent overfilling.

- Keep pocket size wet wipes to hand for emergency changes or wiping the bottom of the bag and your hands, as you may not always have access to water.

- If a leak occurs, try not to panic. Always carry a few pre-cut stoma bags, some wet and dry wipes, rubbish bags, adhesive remover spray/wipes and an extra pair of underwear/clothes for emergency changes. You can leave extra supplies in your car, at work or in a safe place, however, avoid leaving supplies in very high or low temperatures as your stoma products may become damaged. Also check your emergency stock bag to ensure products are still in date.

- If you have a stoma in the **small intestine or your stoma output tends to be high and loose**, you may find it helpful to take Loperamide tablets, and/or add a thickening sachet inside your stoma bag to help thicken the output and prevent leakage.

Use of public toilets – when you have mastered changing and emptying your stoma bag at home you may feel confident to empty or change your bag in a public toilet. Most people find it easier changing their stoma bag in an **accessible toilet**, since there is more space, a washbasin, running water and somewhere to place products. Access to most of these toilets is with a RADAR key which you can purchase online or you can ask your stoma nurse to arrange for you to receive one. Make sure you familiarise yourself with the location of the nearest toilet and know how to access it. There are also some smartphone apps that can navigate you to the nearest toilet.

Ballooning – once you start to eat and drink normally, you may notice that sometimes your stoma bag fills up with air and may even detach from your skin. This is called ballooning. Modern stoma bags are designed with a charcoal filter, which helps release wind and neutralise odour, therefore, preventing ballooning but if the problem persists consider:

- Going to the bathroom and opening your stoma bag to allow the air to exit. If it is a drainable bag, lift the opening upwards and gently press your bag with your hand. If you are using a closed stoma bag you may prefer to use a two-piece system so you can open the seal between the bag and the baseplate.
- If your stoma bag filter gets wet when you shower or swim, use the sticky patches, which come in your stoma box and cover the filter. You must remember to remove the patch afterwards as it will prevent the filter from working.
- Try changing your stoma bag daily instead of every other day so the filter is new.
- Avoid eating in a hurry, skipping meals, chewing gum, talking or drinking while you are eating.
- Avoid food/drinks that cause excessive wind. Use the food charts and tips in this book to remind yourself how to manage wind and what foods/drinks to avoid.

Masking noises – sometimes your stoma may make noises which may be embarrassing at first. Some people find it helpful to cough in order to mask the noise, others may make light of the situation and make a funny comment. Layering your clothes can also muffle the sound from your stoma. The noise from your stoma usually gets less obvious with time.

Letting others know – once you have adjusted to your stoma you may consider whom you would like to tell you have a stoma. It is entirely up to you to decide who should know. Most people would not know that you have a stoma, unless you tell them about it. Your stoma bag is designed to be discreet, not easily visible through your clothing and does not smell unless it is being changed, emptied or is leaking. If you are worried how to talk to people about your stoma, you may want to contact a member of the stoma support group or your stoma nurse for individualised support.

Children – if you have small children and would like to talk about your stoma with them, it may be helpful to invest in a teddy bear with a stoma such as the teddy bear by 'A Bear Named Buttony' charity. These are available to obtain online. Alternatively, you can use the stoma from your practice kit and attach it to any teddy bear or toy you already have at home. If your child is the one that has a stoma, having their favourite toy with a stoma may be an effective way to help them accept their stoma.

Naming your stoma – another effective method for adjustment to life with a stoma, which many people find useful, is giving a name to your stoma. It may be odd for you at first to consider the idea but

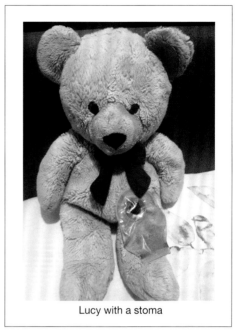

Lucy with a stoma

there are some positive effects of naming your stoma. Naming your stoma can be a discreet way of talking about your stoma in public, if you only want certain people to know about it, may be a helpful way to introduce a stoma to children and loved ones or help with accepting the stoma and bonding with loved ones by choosing a name together.

3. Complications related to stoma formation

Not everyone will develop a complication in hospital or at home following stoma-forming surgery, however, complications with the stoma or peristomal skin are very common and can occur at any time following surgery. Most complications can be easily resolved, **though you may need extra assistance from your stoma nurse or surgical team**.

> **🦁** Developing a stoma complication does not necessarily mean that you are doing your stoma care incorrectly.

Early post-surgery complications (in hospital)

Complications occurring in hospital after surgery are defined as early post-surgery complications and though these complications are not directly related to the stoma, they will have an effect on your stoma function, overall recovery and most likely slow down your stoma care teaching in hospital. If you do develop a complication post-surgery, your stoma nurses will still encourage you to participate in learning how to manage your stoma, as your involvement is vital to ensure your discharge from hospital is not further delayed. Some of the early post-surgery complications are:

Ileus – in order for food and fluid to pass through your intestine, the intestine contracts and relaxes pushing forward the food and fluid, in a process known as peristalsis. When you have surgery peristalsis may slow down and can even stop. This post-surgical complication is known as ileus and is usually caused by the anaesthetic drugs, side effects of some pain medications or handling of the intestine during surgery. Without peristalsis, the food and fluid will not move through your intestine, causing your abdomen to become bloated. You may feel nauseated or start to vomit. Consequently, your stoma will not work or would produce very little output.

What should you do? Try to mobilise as much as possible, as movement may help resolve your ileus. Do not be alarmed as an ileus usually resolves by itself within a few days. Once resolved and your stoma starts working, your stoma output may be erratic and high, therefore you may need a high output stoma bag in order to make stoma management easier for a few days.

Treatment for ileus – in order to help you feel better and relieve the pressure in your abdomen:

- A nasogastric tube may need to be inserted through your nose down your throat and into your stomach. The tube will be secured to your nose with a piece of tape and then a drainage bag will be attached to the other end. This enables the stomach contents to drain into the bag and relieve the bloated feeling and associated nausea.

- You may also need an intravenous drip in order to receive enough fluids and stay hydrated, as you will not be eating and drinking until your ileus resolves.

- If your ileus is due to an obstruction at the level of your stoma such as swelling or kinking (bend) of your intestine, the surgeon or stoma nurse may insert a soft tube (catheter) inside your stoma in order to relieve the pressure. The catheter will need to remain inside until your stoma swelling reduces and it starts to work. You may still be able to participate in stoma teaching with a catheter in the stoma.

Wound infection – the midline wound or one of the port sites (keyholes) can become infected within a few days after your operation and this can make stoma care difficult especially if the wound is near the stoma or under the baseplate.

What should you do? Try not to touch your surgical wounds and keep them clean. Make sure your wound dressings are changed regularly or if they get soiled. Change your stoma bag daily in order to prevent it from leaking onto your wound.

Treatment for wound infection – depending on the nature of your wound infection:

- You may need some of your clips/stitches to be removed earlier than the usual 10 to 14 days post-surgery in order to allow the fluid collected underneath your wound to drain.

- A swab may need to be taken and if you have a confirmed wound infection, your surgeon may suggest a course of antibiotic treatment.

- Developing a wound infection may sometimes interfere with the positioning of your stoma bag, as you may require a dressing on the wound which may obstruct your vision when positioning the stoma bag. You may need extra support or use a mirror to position your bag.

- If the wound is oozing the bag may also lift off, so your stoma nurse can show you how to cut the baseplate 'off centre', to prevent it covering the wound or use a different bag or accessory product to secure it.

> If you have a wound and a dressing, **the stoma bag should be positioned first** to ensure a good seal and where possible, not stuck over the dressing. This will prevent further wound contamination if the stoma bag leaks.

Generally, your stoma nurse will be able to manage a small wound infection, however, if the wound is large and your stoma care is compromised, the stoma nurse may seek advice from the specialist wound care nurse and together they will agree the best plan for managing your wound and stoma. If you are able to go home and the wound has not completely healed, you may be referred to a district nurse or practice nurse to offer you extra support. Once the wound is healed you will be reviewed in a stoma outpatient clinic and shown how to position the stoma bag in the best possible way.

Early stoma and peristomal skin complications

Early complications can occur with the stoma or peristomal skin whilst in hospital or within the first few weeks following surgery. You may be able to self-care and manage most early stoma or peristomal skin complications yourself but your stoma nurse will be on hand to review, manage or treat your stoma complication and if required, teach you how to continue treatment at home. The most common early stoma or peristomal complications are:

Stoma oedema – immediately after surgery, your stoma will be swollen (oedematous). This is normal, as your intestine has been handled during surgery, causing it to become bruised and swollen. It generally takes a couple of days for the swelling to improve, however, your stoma will continue to gradually shrink during the next 4 to 6 weeks as the size and shape becomes more consistent.

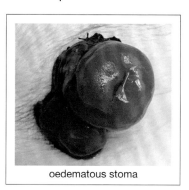

oedematous stoma

What should you do? An oedematous stoma may be more swollen at the top than at the base, like the appearance of a mushroom and therefore it is important to prevent associated skin complications. The baseplate should be cut to the larger size at the top of the stoma and a ring/seal placed around the base of the stoma making sure that the healthy skin is not exposed.

Bleeding – you may notice blood on the wipe when you clean your stoma. This is normal and you should not be alarmed as your stoma has many tiny and delicate blood vessels, which can bleed easily.

What should you do? Make sure you use soft wipes and be gentle while cleaning your stoma, but if you continue to see a bit of blood while wiping and cleaning your stoma, it does not mean that you are doing anything wrong, as it is completely normal. Another reason for your stoma to bleed may be trauma from cutting your stoma baseplate too small and causing injury to the stoma when applying the bag. Make sure you measure your stoma and cut the baseplate correctly.

Treatment for bleeding – apply gentle pressure to the bleeding area and it should usually stop within few minutes. If the bleeding persists, seek medical attention.

> ⚠ If you notice that blood is coming from inside the stoma or the stoma output is red in your bag, seek medical attention immediately.

Mucocutaneous separation (MCS) – occurs when the stoma detaches from the surrounding skin and creates a gap between the stoma and the skin. The separation could be superficial or deep, partial or complete (all around the stoma). This complication is fairly common in the first few weeks after surgery. MCS can also occur when the stitches in your stoma are under excessive tension. Healing may occur spontaneously but depending on the extension and depth of the separation,

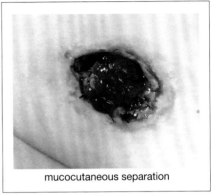

mucocutaneous separation

your stoma nurse may advise treatment. In the absence of treatment complications such as stoma 📖 retraction or 📖 stenosis may occur.

What should you do? Some patients use a mirror to observe the stoma properly or take a daily photograph of the stoma so they can monitor the situation, as it can be difficult to see if the MCS is getting worse, as this process can occur slowly. MCS is usually preceded by the following signs and symptoms, therefore, monitor for these every time you change your stoma bag:

- increased pain around stoma or a dragging sensation when the bag is positioned
- a darker (bruised) discolouration of the peristomal skin
- peristomal skin may appear hot and hard to touch
- very loose or tight stitches
- increased mucus or stoma output on the skin
- stoma appears to be disappearing under the skin

Treatment for MCS – your stoma nurse may need to use accessory products such as stoma powder, Orabase® paste, stoma rings or special dressings, if the separation is deep. When the stoma separates from the skin it may also retract to or below skin level and a convex stoma bag may be required. A convex baseplate applies gentle pressure and raises the stoma above the level of the skin to prevent further skin damage and leakage of the appliance.

> ⚠ Do not use a convex stoma bag without recommendation from your stoma nurse, as convex size and depth varies and incorrect product selection may increase the risk of MCS. You must monitor the surrounding skin for further signs of separation when using a convex bag.

Excoriated (sore) peristomal skin – can occur at any time following surgery and is caused when the skin surrounding your stoma is repeatedly exposed to the stoma output. Your stoma output contains enzymes which break down your food. While these enzymes are useful for your food digestion, they are harmful on your skin.

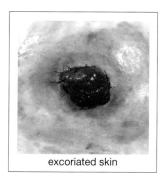

excoriated skin

The most common cause of excoriated skin is due to leakage of an ill-fitting stoma bag but this is usually initiated by a complication occurring with the skin or the stoma.

While an occasional stoma bag leak is considered an accident and should improve as you become more confident, consistent leakage is a concern, as it is a major contributing factor to excoriated skin. There could be several reasons for your skin to become excoriated:

- **Incorrect size of the baseplate** – it is very important to always make sure you are cutting your baseplate to the correct size, allowing a 1–2 mm space between the stoma and the skin. If the hole you are cutting in your baseplate is **too big** your skin will be exposed to the stoma output, therefore it will become excoriated. However, if the hole you are cutting in your baseplate is **too small** your stoma will not be completely surrounded by the stoma baseplate and leakage occurs underneath the baseplate.

  What should you do? You should measure your stoma twice weekly in the first 6 weeks following stoma-forming surgery and regularly if you notice changes with your weight or abdominal girth, in order to ensure a good fit.

- **Irregular abdominal contours** – changes in body shape such as weight gain or loss, illnesses causing abdominal bloating, pregnancy and scarring from previous surgery, may result in the skin forming creases, dips or folds which prevent the stoma bag forming a tight seal with the skin. Stoma care may also become more challenging which in itself can continue to exacerbate the problem.

  What should you do? Use a mirror or ask someone to help you correctly position the stoma bag. If this does not help contact your stoma nurse for further advice as you may need to use a different stoma bag or add accessories.

- **Rapid removal of your stoma bag** – some people may have delicate or sensitive skin which is prone to damage if the stoma bag is rapidly pulled off the skin.

  What should you do? A remover spray can be helpful to remove the used stoma bag but you can also remove the bag without an adhesive remover if you stretch the skin slightly and slowly lift the bag off the skin. A remover spray should be used sparingly, allowing time for the spray to drip down under the baseplate before pulling the bag off.

- **Over-cleaning** – it is possible to over cleanse the skin or cause damage by using harsh cleaning products or wipes.

  What should you do? Warm tap water and soft cleaning wipes are sufficient to remove stoma output from the skin. Some people can clean their stoma whilst in the shower as long as direct water pressure is not used on the stoma. There is no need for soap or disinfectant wipes.

- **More liquid or higher stoma output** – liquid output can flow easier than formed output underneath the baseplate of your stoma bag and irritate your skin or cause the stoma bag to leak. You may not even be aware that this is happening. This process can make skin sore within hours, especially if you are emptying your bag more frequently because the output is also higher than usual.

  What should you do? You will need to check regularly to ensure your stoma bag is attached to your skin and if it shows signs of leakage change it as soon as possible. If the watery output persists for more than 48 hours, you may need to contact your stoma nurse as you may need to take medication to help thicken and slow down your output, as well as, make some changes to your diet. A diet high in carbohydrates but low in fibre will help thicken your output.

>   Care must be taken when making dietary changes, especially if you have underlying health conditions. You should not stop eating unless advised to, as this can make a liquid, high output worse.

- **Delayed stoma bag change** – it is advisable to change your stoma bag every 1–3 days, depending on the type of stoma you have or the output produced. If you wait for the bag to leak before you change it, then you will be more likely to experience excoriated skin.

  What should you do? Everyone is different and it will be up to you to learn what works best for you. A good rule of thumb is to start changing your stoma bag every day and if the peristomal skin looks healthy and you are not experiencing any leakage, try changing your bag every other day or every two days. However, if you notice that your skin starts to look red and irritated or you start experiencing leakage between bag changes, it is best to go back to changing your stoma bag more regularly. If you require help to change your stoma bag, it is better to change it more frequently than to have the bag leak and then wait for assistance.

Treatment for excoriated skin – your stoma nurse has the knowledge and products available to treat your skin excoriation. Depending on the level of severity, your stoma nurse may need to use a combination of stoma accessories such as stoma powder, paste or rings or ultimately use a different stoma bag.

> 🐾 Once your skin has healed you will not need to use stoma accessory products. Do not dispose of excess stock in case you need them in the future **but remind your GP, prescribing hub or DAC to remove them from your monthly prescription.**

Stoma necrosis – if the blood supply to your stoma is obstructed or interrupted, stoma necrosis or 'tissue death' may occur. A necrotic stoma can appear flaccid or hard but will be discoloured, dusky and dry, rather than red and moist. It may be purple, brown or black in colour and usually occurs immediately after surgery or within the first 5 days after surgery. Necrosis may be superficial or deep and may cover the entire surface of the stoma or appear in patches. Common reasons for stoma necrosis could be:

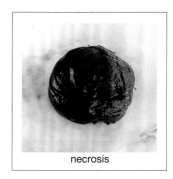

necrosis

- excessive stretching of the intestine and its blood vessels
- very swollen or oedematous intestine after surgery
- insufficient blood supply to the intestine because of a thick abdominal wall caused by swelling of the abdomen, distention or obesity
- very close or overly tight stitches around the stoma causing tissue damage
- excessive pressure from your stoma baseplate opening when the hole is cut too small

What should you do? Contact your stoma nurse or surgeon.

Treatment for necrosis – your stoma nurse or your surgeon will need to inspect your stoma by inserting either a lubricated finger into the stoma or a small test tube with a light to inspect the intestine behind the stoma and determine the level of necrosis. If the stoma necrosis is limited to the superficial portion of the intestine above the abdominal skin level, management is conservative but closely monitored. The superficial dead tissue will slowly come off and healthy tissue will begin to show. During this period your stoma nurse would use a clear stoma bag so that nursing and medical staff can monitor the colour of your stoma. As your stoma heals and the dead tissue continues to fall off, your stoma may slightly retract below or at the level of your skin or its opening may become stenosed or narrowed and you may need help stretching it. Your stoma nurse would help you manage those complications as additional stoma accessories may be required. If the necrosis expands further down the intestine below the abdominal surface, then you will need to go back to surgery immediately. Your surgeon will need to remove the portion of necrotic intestine and refashion your stoma.

Late stoma and peristomal skin complications

Late stoma or peristomal skin complications can occur months or even years following surgery and it is unlikely that you will be able to manage these complications by yourself, however, your stoma nurse will be on hand to assist. You may be asked to provide some details about your operation and stoma so it is helpful to have this information to hand before speaking to your stoma nurse. However, if your problem persists and you and your stoma nurse are unable to find a solution, you may need to have a surgical opinion to refashion your stoma leaving it at the same site, or the stoma may be moved to another position. The most common late stoma or peristomal complications are:

Stoma obstruction – you will now have a routine for when your stoma works and when it is more or less active. However, if your stoma has not been as active in the day as it usually is and your abdomen becomes bloated or you experience abdominal cramps or nausea and vomiting, you may have an obstruction. A stoma obstruction may occur at any time and it is commonly caused by undigested food (food bolus) that obstructs the faecal flow. It can also be caused by inflammation, trauma, swelling, narrowing, scarring or a bend/twist in the intestine above the stoma. **Appendix 3 details St Mark's Hospital guide to managing stoma obstruction**.

Your stoma obstruction may be **complete** when no output comes out or **partial** when some watery output may continue to pass. The watery output may be green or yellow in colour, which is mainly bile.

It is normal to see bile in your stoma bag if the stoma is blocked and the bile is not mixed with stool, especially with a stoma in the small intestine, or if you have not eaten for a long period of time. Bile may also cause an unpleasant or unusual odour when emptying the stoma bag.

> A stoma obstruction is usually managed by keeping you comfortable and giving your body time to resolve the obstruction on its own, using the methods mentioned below. **Surgery is not the first line of treatment for stoma obstruction.**

What should you do? It is common for the stoma obstruction to self-resolve but if that does not happen, try the following steps over **a couple of hours**:

- stop eating food and only drink clear fluids like water, tea, vegetable/meat stock
- if you are not nauseated or vomiting, try drinking 1–2 glasses of water quickly as sometimes drinking fluids quickly may help flush the food bolus out
- try massaging your abdomen around the stoma
- try changing position such as pulling your knees up to your chest or rolling from one side to another
- a warm bath may help relax your abdominal muscles
- try putting a hot water bottle on your abdomen which also helps manage associated pain
- light exercise such as walking may encourage the intestine to move more
- you may need to cut the opening of your stoma baseplate a bit larger than usual as your stoma may increase in size and become swollen
- do not be tempted to take laxatives unless advised by a healthcare professional

> ⚠ If your stoma is still not working and you are feeling more nauseated or continue to vomit and the abdominal cramps do not resolve or become worse, seek urgent medical attention.

Treatment for stoma obstruction – in the emergency department, the medical staff will help you with your obstructive symptoms. You may need an intravenous drip to make sure you stay hydrated as you would not be eating or drinking. Some scans may be done to confirm whether you have an obstruction and pain relief should be given to you to help with your discomfort.

If a stoma obstruction is confirmed, you may have to refrain from eating and drinking until the obstruction resolves. A tube may be inserted through your nose and passed down your throat all the way to your stomach. This helps relieve nausea and vomiting. A soft tube (catheter) may be inserted inside your stoma to decompress your abdomen and help treat your abdominal distention.

The catheter will need to remain inside until your stoma obstruction resolves and it starts to work. If the scan confirms the cause of the obstruction to **not** be a food bolus, you may need an operation to resolve the problem.

> Remember to take your stoma wash bag with you if you go to hospital to ensure that you have everything you need, as it may be difficult to find your exact stoma products, especially out of hours, on weekends or bank holidays.

Dehydration – having a stoma may put you at higher risk of becoming dehydrated, especially if you have a **small intestine stoma**, as part of your intestine no longer takes part of your digestion and you tend to lose more fluid, salt and nutrients. Having a stoma does not necessarily mean that you would become dehydrated, however, there are several reasons that may lead to dehydration:

- **High output stoma** – having a high output can quickly lead to dehydration. When you notice that your stoma output is rather loose and you empty your stoma bag more often than usual, you most likely are experiencing a high output. Try to think of possible reasons for your high output stoma. Have you had any food/drinks that may have upset your stomach or food/drinks you do not usually tolerate well? Have you travelled abroad recently and possibly picked up an infection? Have you gone out for a meal which has led to food poisoning or eaten raw or undercooked food? Have you taken antibiotics, laxatives or medications that may cause diarrhoea as a side effect? It is always important to find out the cause for your high output stoma, because usually you may improve your symptoms by simply eliminating the reason for it.

- **Vomiting** – you are at risk of dehydration if you are vomiting, caused by extra fluid loss. If you are unable to keep your fluids down and you continue to vomit, you may need to go to the hospital to have intravenous fluids to replace your fluid losses.

- **Hot weather and excessive sweating** – you lose minerals and salts through sweat therefore you will need to replace these losses.

- **Excessive physical activities, exercise and sports** – may cause dehydration due to excessive sweating and lack of hydration when concentrating or involved in competitive sports.

- **Travelling** – you may become dehydrated when travelling as you alter your daily routines, sleep patterns or even cross different time zones, making it difficult to keep track of your fluid intake or requirements.

- **Stoma obstruction** – can lead to dehydration if you are unable to eat or drink or the obstruction causes repeated episodes of vomiting.

Signs and symptoms of dehydration	
Feeling lightheaded or dizzy	Concentrated, dark coloured and smelly urine
Headaches – especially when you stand up quickly	Passing urine less often than usual
Feeling thirsty despite drinking	Dark sunken eyes
Dry lips and mouth	Muscle cramps
Dry skin	Weak or rapid pulse
Sudden weight loss	Fits (seizures)
Low energy and feeling tired	Becoming drowsy or unresponsive

What should you do? It is best to **prevent dehydration** rather than having to treat it, therefore if you notice that your stoma output becomes very watery or green in colour and increases in volume, you should:

- avoid diuretic drinks such as caffeinated tea, coffee and cola
- avoid drinking too much alcohol
- avoid sugar-free food/drinks containing xylitol, sorbitol or mannitol
- keep yourself hydrated and drink 1.5–2 litres or 8–10 glasses of fluids a day
- eat foods rich in water such as melon, yoghurt and cottage cheese
- eat foods that thicken your output
- carry a bottle and sip fluids throughout the day
- drink **slightly** more fluids in the case of hot weather, increased physical activity or excessive sweating but do not drink in excess of 3–4 litres
- drink sport drinks like Gatorade®, Lucozade® or Powerade® or rehydrating drinks like St Mark's E–mix solution or Dioralyte™
- avoid drinking fluids too quickly as this may 'flush' the fluid out your intestine and result in further losses
- monitor your urine colour – your urine should be a clear or light yellow colour when you are well hydrated and dark and concentrated when you are becoming dehydrated

- monitor urine output – when your body is becoming dehydrated it starts producing less urine, therefore, you will pass urine less often

Treatment for dehydration – severe dehydration is usually treated by administering intravenous fluids, monitoring urine and stoma output and testing urine and blood levels.

Granulomas – sometimes you may notice small, red lumps on or around your stoma, especially where the stoma joins the skin. They may develop as a result of prolonged inflammation from stoma output being in contact with your skin, irritation from stitches or possibly due to friction from the bag or clothing. Some granulomas can cause bleeding and discomfort, while others do not cause any problems.

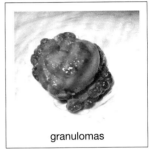

granulomas

What should you do? Be gentle when cleaning and drying the stoma to prevent further bleeding or trauma. Make sure that you cut the baseplate to the correct size to avoid friction and if possible, **fit the baseplate to cover the granulomas**.

Treatment for granulomas – sometimes removing stoma stitches may reduce granuloma formation. If your granulomas get bigger and cause your bag to leak or become painful, your stoma nurse may need to treat them over a few weeks using a Silver Nitrate 75% preparation or Fludroxycortide (Haelan® tape). Your stoma nurse may advise you to use a softer stoma baseplate, stoma rings/seals or paste to reduce friction and help with the healing process. If your granulomas are too big or do not respond to treatment you may need a minor surgical procedure to have them removed.

> ⚠️ If you are allergic to silver, remember to inform your stoma nurse, as Silver Nitrate treatment may cause an allergic reaction.

Stoma prolapse – a portion of your intestine may move outside your abdomen through your stoma opening, known as a stoma prolapse.

A stoma prolapse can occur in any type of stoma, however, it is more commonly seen with loop stomas and in particular with a loop colostomy.

A prolapsed stoma would increase both in width and in length. Stoma prolapse usually occurs in the following situations:

- if your stoma is not adequately fixed to your abdominal wall during your surgery, causing the intestine to slide through the stoma opening

- weak abdominal muscles
- when your stoma is not created within your abdominal rectus muscle
- increased pressure inside your abdomen, e.g. coughing, sneezing, vomiting
- obesity
- pregnancy
- in the presence of a parastomal hernia

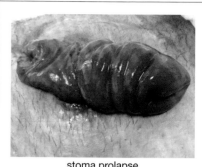

stoma prolapse

What should you do? Protect your stoma from trauma and bleeding by using a stoma shield or a hernia support belt to prevent more of the intestine from sliding through the stoma opening. You should sleep on your back or side as sleeping on your abdomen may damage the prolapsed intestine. You may need to use a larger and longer stoma bag to accommodate the intestine inside the bag. Your stoma nurse may suggest making tiny slits around the inner edge of the stoma baseplate opening to allow for the prolapsed intestine to move freely.

> Only apply a support belt or stoma shield once the prolapsed intestine is reduced back inside your abdomen and while you are lying flat.

Apply a cold compress or sugar to the stoma for 5–10 minutes to help reduce swelling and make it easier for the stoma prolapse to slide back in. You may need to resize your baseplate opening and make it larger as the prolapse will cause your stoma to change shape. A larger baseplate opening would expose your peristomal skin to stoma output, so you may also require stoma seals/rings around the exposed peristomal skin to prevent excoriation.

Your prolapsed stoma may lead to an obstruction, so you should monitor for the following signs and symptoms:

- abdominal cramps and pain
- nausea and/or vomiting
- bloated or distended abdomen
- no stoma output or decreased stoma output

Treatment for a stoma prolapse – with the help of your stoma nurse you should be able to manage your stoma prolapse conservatively and your stoma nurse will be able to teach you how to manually reduce the prolapse

If you notice that your stoma stops working or changes colour and becomes darker, paler or dusky **seek urgent medical attention**, as this may mean that your intestine is being strangulated and the blood supply is limited.

back inside your abdomen while lying flat on your back and applying continuous gentle pressure to the intestine. Many people live with a prolapsed stoma without any concerns. However, if your stoma prolapse continues to cause you discomfort you may need to consult your surgeon for surgical repair and refashioning of the stoma.

 Do not try to reduce your prolapse without being trained by your stoma nurse as an incorrect technique may make the situation worse.

Retraction – if your stoma is under tension when fashioned it can retract into your abdomen especially when the initial swelling reduces.

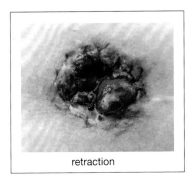
retraction

If this happens your stoma bag may start to leak frequently or you may experience skin irritation, as the stoma output will be draining onto your skin under the bag. Anyone with a stoma can experience retraction. Your stoma may retract entirely/circumferentially or partly.

The following reasons increase the risk for your stoma to retract:

- if you gain an excessive amount of weight after your surgery
- an insufficient length of intestine to form your stoma during surgery
- early removal of supporting device (bridge/rod) in loop stoma
- poor fixation of your stoma to your abdomen
- early removal of stoma stitches
- as a result of mucocutaneous separation
- if you have Crohn's disease
- steroid and immunosuppressant use
- malnutrition

What should you do? Contact your stoma nurse to review the stoma. Try to lose weight if possible, if this is the reason for your stoma retraction. Stoma retraction is usually managed with the use of stoma accessories or changing your stoma bag to one with a convex baseplate and/or using a stoma belt to better secure the appliance and help prevent leakage.

Treatment for stoma retraction – a retracted stoma is at risk of becoming narrow and your stoma nurse may need to use an instrument called a stoma dilator to prevent your retracted stoma opening from becoming too small.

Stenosis – is characterised by a narrowing of your stoma opening or the intestine just behind the opening which may prevent proper drainage of stoma output. You may get easily bloated, experience abdominal pain and cramping, diarrhoea, increased wind and feel nauseated or vomit, after meals. You may notice that the stoma output reduces, becomes more difficult to pass or stops completely, which is referred to as a 📖 stoma obstruction.

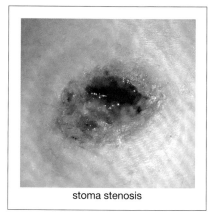

stoma stenosis

Stenosis can be due to associated scar tissue restricting the opening of the stoma, especially if you have been treated recently for stoma retraction, mucocutaneous separation or a degree of necrosis or infection around the stoma.

If the surgical incision in the abdomen is too small or the abdominal muscle is too tight, you can experience symptoms related to stenosis as the narrowing may be behind the stoma in the abdomen. Treatments such as radiotherapy can also cause stenosis.

Urostomy stenosis – stenosis may occur in any stoma, which includes a urostomy. A healthy urostomy should constantly produce urine, so monitor for possible signs and symptoms of stenosis such as stoma bag leakage, excoriated skin, decreased urine output, flank pain or recurrent urinary infections.

What should you do? Contact your stoma nurse as a stenosed stoma puts you at a higher risk of a 📖 stoma obstruction. You should therefore try to eat a soft, low fibre diet, increase your fluid intake or use laxatives and stool softeners, if appropriate for your type of stoma.

Treatment for stenosis – your stoma nurse will provide diet and lifestyle advice specific to your requirements. They may also need to teach you how to use an instrument called a dilator in order to keep your stoma open.

If the dilator is not helping to keep the stoma open, you may need to have surgery. During your operation, your surgeon will refashion your stoma and leave it at the same site or move it elsewhere on your abdomen.

Parastomal hernia – during your stoma formation an incision is made through your abdomen in order to bring your stoma through. The incision weakens your abdominal muscles, putting you at higher risk of developing a hernia. A parastomal hernia, is a bulging of your intestine under the peristomal skin. The bulge may reduce back inside your abdomen when you are lying flat and reappear when you are standing. A parastomal hernia may occur in any type of stoma, but is more common in people with a loop colostomy or a double-barrel stoma.

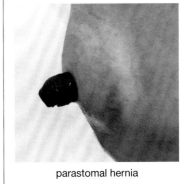
parastomal hernia

The risk of developing a parastomal hernia is higher in the first few weeks after your surgery, however, you can develop a parastomal hernia any time after your surgery. Most people experience pain and discomfort as the hernia gets bigger and describe a sensation of heaviness or dragging around the stoma.

Parastomal hernia predisposing factors		
Increased age	Malnutrition	Stoma formation outside the rectus muscle
Multiple operations	Wide abdominal defect	
Wound infections	Peristomal infection	Poor abdominal wall support
Heavy lifting	Diminished muscle tone	
Obesity		Increased abdominal pressure – coughing, sneezing, vomiting
Steroid therapy	Collagen defects/ disorder	
Smoking	Construction defects	
Loop stoma	Pregnancy	
Double-barrel stoma		

A parastomal hernia may lead to a 📖 stoma obstruction or your parastomal hernia may become **strangulated**, if the herniated intestine becomes trapped between the abdominal muscles, interrupting the blood supply to your intestine. A strangulated hernia is an emergency as it may lead to death of your intestinal tissue. The following are signs and symptoms of strangulated hernia:

- nausea and/or vomiting
- sudden pain that quickly becomes severe
- stoma stops working or output reduces
- hernia bulge that turns red, purple or dark in colour
- your stoma may become dusky, black or necrotic

> ⚠ If you suspect a strangulated hernia, seek medical attention immediately.

What should you do? Contact your stoma nurse as they will be able to advise you on how to best manage your parastomal hernia. If you experience leakage from the stoma bag you may need a different type of stoma bag and/or a stoma belt. There are modern stoma bags with a concave baseplate that is designed to fit snugly around the bulge and prevent leakage. Alternatively, your stoma nurse may consider using a bag with a larger baseplate as this should provide better adherence. Your stoma nurse may suggest you use flange extenders/security frames around the baseplate to prolong wear time. A parastomal hernia may also stretch your peristomal skin making it thinner and more fragile, therefore, it is important to take extra care when removing your baseplate especially if you use extra flange extenders, as damage to your skin may occur.

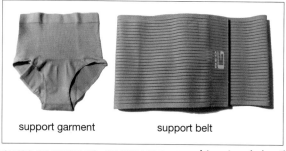

support garment   support belt

The pressure created by the parastomal hernia may change the shape of your stoma, therefore, make sure you measure your stoma regularly and resize your baseplate accordingly. If you have colostomy and irrigate, speak to your stoma nurse or surgeon, as you may need to stop irrigating as the hernia may restrict the flow of water into and out of your stoma.

Support garments and belts are used to either prevent or relieve the symptoms of a parastomal hernia, bulging abdomen or an odd abdominal shape. Your stoma nurse will be able to advise you on a range of support garments and belts to help you support the weight of the hernia and relieve the dragging sensation when you are active.

Apply your belt while lying flat on your back and only when your hernia has been reduced back into your abdominal cavity. Wear your belt when walking and doing exercise, lifting or sports and remove it when you are asleep or relaxing.

A wide range of support garments and belts are available on prescription or for you to buy. You should only order one belt in the first instance to ensure it fits comfortably and that you can tolerate wearing it.

> It is strongly recommended that you have a fitting by an experienced healthcare professional, as you may need a bespoke garment and your measurements must be accurate.

Treatment for a parastomal hernia – usually people manage to live with their parastomal hernia, however, if your parastomal hernia is causing you too much discomfort and is interfering with your daily life, you may need to have an operation. Your surgeon will repair your hernia and may need to refashion your stoma and leave it at the same site, or move it elsewhere on your abdomen, if necessary.

Prevention of parastomal hernia

- Wear a hernia support belt if you are at risk of developing a hernia

- Support your abdomen with your hand or a small cushion when coughing, sneezing or vomiting as these actions increase the pressure inside your abdomen and strain your abdominal muscles.

- Avoid lifting anything heavier than 2.5 kg (5 lb) for the first 8–12 weeks after your surgery. The following everyday household items are approximately 2 kg – a kettle, 2-litre bottle of water, a casserole or a small laundry basket. Avoid carrying shopping bags and try to refrain from lifting children or pets.

- Avoid activities at home such as gardening, moving furniture, vacuuming or pushing a pram, wheelchair or shopping trolley, for the first 8–12 weeks after your surgery.

- Smoking is a known risk for parastomal hernia development. It is highly advisable that you try to seek help to stop smoking.

- Exercising and strengthening your core abdominal muscles, **before** your surgery can be helpful to prevent a parastomal hernia. Any exercise meant to build up your abdominal muscles is good enough but do not pressure yourself to exercise if you are not used to doing so. Two weeks **after your surgery**, you can start light exercise, such as walking and gradually increasing the time and intensity as you feel ready. Avoid straining and lifting weights. Once you have returned to your normal routines, speak with your stoma nurse who can advise if you require extra abdominal support wear.

Allergy – in rare cases, you may develop an allergy to the baseplate, stoma bag or any of the stoma accessory products. The peristomal skin can become dry, damp or itchy and a red area develops in the shape of the bag, baseplate or accessory on your skin.

What should you do? Contact your stoma nurse as you will not be able to manage a true allergy yourself.

Treatment for allergy – you may need an allergy patch test with different stoma products in order to

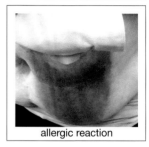

allergic reaction

determine if you have an allergy and the products you are allergic to. Your stoma nurse will help you choose a different system if this is the case. In very rare cases you may be allergic to a wide range of stoma bags and/or accessories, therefore, you will be referred to a dermatologist for further investigations.

> ⚠ Once it has been confirmed which products you are allergic to, you must remember not to use them again and inform your stoma nurse.

Pyoderma gangrenosum (PG) – is a rare condition that causes extremely painful pustules or ulcers to develop on your skin, most often on your legs, but also around your peristomal skin. It is believed to be a disorder of your immune system.

Patients with a history of inflammatory bowel disease or arthritis are at higher risk of having PG with typical red open ulcers with a purple or blue coloured well-defined border. The ulcer edges are irregular and the surrounding skin is red and hard to touch.

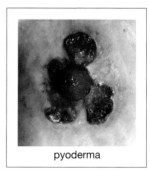

pyoderma

What should you do? Contact your stoma nurse as you will not be able to manage PG without medical intervention.

Treatment for PG – PG needs to be diagnosed by your stoma nurse or surgeon as soon as possible, as you will need to use topical or oral corticosteroids and/or immunosuppressant medication in order to treat PG. Unfortunately, PG may take time to heal and it may also reappear in the future.

Folliculitis – if you have excessive amount of hair on the skin around your stoma, it may prevent the bag from sticking or shorten the wear time and cause leakage. Some people choose to shave the area around their stoma in order to achieve better adhesion of their stoma bag and less traumatic removal of their used stoma bag. While shaving the area around the stoma is effective, it may cause an infection in the hair follicles known as folliculitis. Folliculitis is characterised by a red rash with tiny white-headed pimples over the shaved area.

What should you do? Use an electric trimmer rather than a razor or hair remover products, as these could irritate your skin. If you decide to use a razor, remember to use one without lubricating strips, as these may leave an oily residue on the skin which may prevent the stoma bag from sticking. Shave your skin once a week or as needed. Try not to shave too often. Do not be tempted to use lotion or creams on your skin as this may prevent the stoma bag sticking.

Treatment for folliculitis – keep the area clean and dry. Avoid shaving the area for a few weeks. The use of a mild antibacterial soap may also be effective. Sometimes topical antibiotics may be required and if this is the case it is better to use a cream than an ointment to ensure your stoma bag adheres properly.

Stoma laceration – is described as a 'cut' or 'tear' in the stoma mucosa and usually occurs as a result of accidental trauma. Unless there is obvious bleeding, you may not even notice small lacerations or feel any pain in the stoma. Most lacerations usually heal once you remove the cause. The most common causes of lacerations are shaving injuries, the result of improper sizing of your baseplate, sporting injuries and rough clothing or a belt which comes in regular contact with your stoma. It is rare that you will need surgery unless the trauma is major or the bleeding does not stop easily.

What should you do? If actively bleeding, apply direct pressure to the laceration for a few minutes until the bleeding stops. If bleeding is not of concern and the laceration was caused by:

- **Clothing or a belt** – try positioning your belt above or below your stoma and not on top of it. You may even benefit from wearing braces or altering your waistband and wearing loose fitting clothes.
- **Shaving** – in order to protect your stoma and avoid any unintentional cuts while shaving the surrounding skin you can use an empty toilet paper roll to put over the stoma. You should also shave the hair on your peristomal skin in the direction away from your stoma.
- **Sport** – avoid contact sports or speak to your stoma nurse and they will provide suitable lifestyle advice. You may also benefit from a stoma shield to protect the stoma.
- **Baseplate or template trauma** – resize the stoma carefully, especially if you use a hard, plastic measuring guide or speak to your stoma nurse who can resize the stoma and provide the correct template.

Treatment for a stoma laceration – depending on how serious the laceration of your stoma is, you may need stitches placed in the stoma or cauterisation of the bleeding blood vessel.

 If the bleeding does not stop, **seek urgent medical attention** as the injury to your stoma may be more serious than it appears.

Non-stoma related surgical complications

After your stoma surgery you may experience complications which are not related to the stoma but worth mentioning to your stoma nurse or surgeon if you are concerned.

Rectal discharge – if your rectum and anus are preserved following your stoma surgery, you may occasionally experience a discharge coming from your anus (back passage). This is normal as the lining of your rectum produces a lubricant called **mucus** which usually mixes with the faeces making movement through the intestine easier. Without faeces coming into the rectum, the mucus is not removed and can build up and therefore leak from your anus.

The frequency and amount of rectal discharge varies depending on the individual and can be passed multiple times a day or on a weekly or monthly basis. Some people report reduction of the rectal discharge with time but this is not always the case and it is unlikely to stop completely. Normal rectal discharge is relatively odourless, clear or white in colour with a sticky glue-like consistency and should pass through your anus easily. Alternatively, it could be passed as a hard ball if the discharge builds up before it is expelled. Sometimes the mucus may be a beige, light brown or dark brown colour in the first few weeks after surgery, as the mucus may be mixed with old blood and faeces left behind in the rectum after your surgery.

If you have a **loop stoma** the mucus may be stained with faeces, therefore the colour may be similar to the colour of your stoma output. You may not always be aware that you need to evacuate the mucus and unfortunately it may leak from your anus.

 If your surgeon closes your back passage and removes your rectum and anus, you will **not** experience rectal discharge. However, if there is a discharge post-surgery you may have a **wound infection** and will need to be seen by your surgeon.

What should you do? Even though it could be frustrating having to deal with rectal discharge, you will need to learn to live with it unless it becomes problematic.

- Some people find pads or panty liners to be helpful especially when going out, as it offers extra protection against leaks onto your underwear.

- Rectal discharge can cause sore skin around your anus. Good perianal care should be performed regularly by washing the area carefully with warm water from a showerhead or in a bath, dab dry the skin well and applying an effective barrier cream. Use water-based, alcohol-free wet wipes when away from home and apply small amount of barrier cream when necessary.

- You may find it helpful to sit on the toilet daily for a few minutes to allow for mucus to be evacuated and reduce the risk of mucus build-up.

- If you cannot control the discharge, pelvic floor exercises may help you tone your anal muscles and control leakage.

> ⚠ If the mucus is bright red, black, greenish or yellow in colour and is accompanied by an unpleasant smell, **seek urgent medical attention**, as this may be a sign of infection, inflammation or tissue damage.

Treatment for rectal discharge – there are some techniques your stoma nurse or surgeon may suggest as treatment.

- Sometimes it is difficult to eliminate the build-up of mucus, which can harden and cause discomfort. **Glycerine 4 g suppositories** could be used as recommended and can be prescribed by your GP or by some stoma nurses.

- Some people may benefit from a **distal washout** which helps flush the build-up of mucus. You can discuss with your stoma nurse to see if this is suitable for you.

- If all suggested techniques do not help, a surgical review will be arranged to decide if removing the rectum and anus (back passage) is in your best interest.

Phantom rectum syndrome – if your stoma surgery involved removal of your rectum and anus (back passage) with the surgical closure of your anus, you may still feel the sensation of rectal fullness and the need to open your bowels through your back passage like you used to do before your operation.

This is described as phantom rectum syndrome. It is a common phenomenon for many people and they may also report pressure or pain in their perineum (bottom) and a tingling, stinging or burning sensation. The sensation usually disappears with time, but some people continue to experience problems long term.

What should you do? The best way to deal with this problem is to sit for a few minutes on the toilet just as you used to do before you had your rectum and anus removed. This usually helps relieve the feeling to open your bowel.

Treatment for phantom rectum syndrome – if conservative treatment does not help, your stoma nurse or surgeon may consider neuropathic pain medications, clinical hypnotherapy or alternative medicine.

Sexual dysfunction – after your stoma operation it is common to experience a loss of libido (reduced sex drive), however, if your rectum is partially or fully removed or your bladder removed during surgery, you may experience some form of sexual dysfunction. In men, problems such as erectile dysfunction (inability to achieve or maintain an erection) or ejaculatory problems (such as retrograde ejaculation) may occur. Women may experience symptoms which cause painful intercourse (dyspareunia). However these problems are usually temporary and resolve within a few months after your surgery.

What should you do? Speak to your partner, stoma nurse or surgeon if you are experiencing any of these problems.

Treatment for sexual dysfunction – you may need to be referred to a specialist urologist or a gynaecologist who will be able to help you with any prolonged sexual problems. Sperm banking or egg harvesting may be options to consider if there is going to be considerable damage during surgery to the prostrate or seminal vesicles in men, scaring around the fallopian tubes in women or if chemotherapy/radiotherapy is required as part of your treatment.

> ⚠ **Before** undergoing stoma-forming surgery it is important to discuss your risk of sexual dysfunction or reduced fertility, especially in people of childbearing age.

Enterocutaneous fistula (ECF) – is an abnormal communication between your gastrointestinal tract and the skin which allows faecal matter to escape from the intestine. There are many reasons why an ECF may develop, but it usually thrives in what is known as a 'hostile abdomen'. Patients who have had multiple abdominal operations, a history of a leak or sepsis in an area where the intestine was previously joined or an

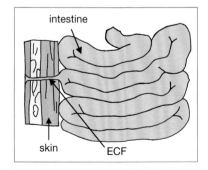

underlying diagnosis of inflammatory bowel disease, can create a hostile abdomen. Other reasons for ECF to develop could be trauma to the abdomen and internal organs, diverticular disease, cancer and consequences of radiotherapy. The faecal output from an ECF could vary from up to 200 ml a day to over 1500–3000 ml, depending on how much intestine you have. Managing an ECF can be a challenging task, involving the support of many healthcare professionals. You may need a stoma nurse, colorectal surgeons, gastroenterologists, dietitians and nutrition nurses who will be able to plan the best management for your ECF.

If your ECF produces a high output, you will not only lose fluids, but also important nutrients and electrolytes, leading to dehydration and malnutrition. **The Lennard Jones Intestinal Rehabilitation Unit** at St Mark's Hospital, is a world-renowned specialist centre dedicated to the assessment and management of patients with intestinal failure and enterocutaneous fistulae. Therefore, these highly trained healthcare professionals will be able to help you become as independent as possible to care for your ECF, if management is conservative or prepare you for an operation, if your ECF is planned for surgical repair.

What should you do? If the ECF is not very large, stoma bags may be sufficient to contain the fistula or if the ECF is larger, an appliance called a wound manager (fistula bag) will be used. In addition, your stoma nurse may need to use stoma accessories such as stoma rings/seals, stoma paste, powder and flange extenders. If you are well enough, your stoma nurse will teach you how to manage your ECF independently.

However, if you cannot care for your ECF yourself, your stoma nurse may need to teach a member of your family who will be able to care for it daily. If your GP considers that it will be appropriate for you to have a package of care with someone to come and visit you at least once a day, this person could be trained by the community stoma nurse, if appropriate. Alternatively, if you have your own private carers, who are willing to care for your ECF, they could be trained by your stoma nurse before you are discharged from the hospital. However, if the management of your ECF is too complex a district nurse may need to visit you at home for ECF management. Before your discharge home your stoma nurses will create a photographic or video step-by-step care plan, with your consent, in order to facilitate your complex ECF management for your district nurses or carers.

Treatment for ECF – some ECF heal on their own, with the correct nutritional and medical input, while more complex ECF require surgery in order to repair or resect the fistula and repair the abdominal wall. You may also require a stoma in order to allow the intestine to heal or if a large section of intestine needs to be removed.

4. Ileostomy

Each year approximately 9,000 new patients[2] in the UK undergo ileostomy formation. This figure includes patients with either a permanent or temporary ileostomy.

On average, an ileostomy produces around 600–800 ml per day of a semi-liquid (porridge-like) or liquid output, however, it is not uncommon for a normal output to range up to 1200 ml per day.

An ileostomy is usually formed on the right side of your abdomen, though this is not always the case and will depend on your personal circumstances, anatomy and other pre-existing medical conditions. An ileostomy may be formed as an end, loop or double-barrel stoma.

Types of operations that may require an ileostomy

☐ Total / Subtotal colectomy

Both of these operations are almost identical, the difference is that during **total colectomy** all of your colon is removed, while during **subtotal colectomy** the last part of your colon remains. In both cases your rectum and anus (back passage) remain in place and an **end ileostomy** is formed. The remaining colon and rectum may either be sewn up and left inside your abdomen or brought out through your abdomen as a second stoma, called a **mucous fistula**.

A mucous fistula may be brought out in your pelvic region or next to your ileostomy. **The rectum will continue to produce mucus and you may experience a mucus discharge from your anus**.

At later stage you may have a second operation to remove your remaining colon, rectum and anus and keep your end ileostomy permanently (panproctocolectomy) or alternatively you may be a candidate for an ileoanal pouch.

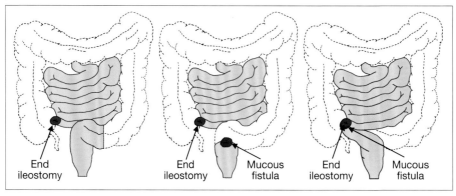

End ileostomy

End ileostomy   Mucous fistula

End ileostomy   Mucous fistula

Panproctocolectomy

The colon, rectum and anus are removed during surgery and your back passage will be stitched closed. A **permanent end ileostomy** is formed.

Sometimes you may develop a breakdown of the wound in the area that was stitched closed and therefore it is important to avoid sitting on your bottom for too long and ensuring the perianal area is kept clean and dry.

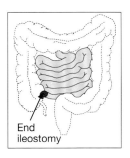

End ileostomy

Ileoanal pouch

The colon and rectum are removed and a reservoir (pouch) is fashioned from part of your small intestine.

The pouch is then joined onto the anus and a **temporary loop ileostomy** is fashioned above the pouch. The loop ileostomy can be reversed in a separate operation.

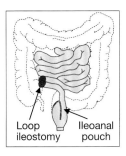

Loop ileostomy   Ileoanal pouch

Low anterior resection of rectum/Total Mesorectal Excision (TME)

The two operations are almost identical. In both cases the last part of your colon (sigmoid) and **almost all** of your rectum will be removed. The difference is that during **total mesorectal excision**, the **lymph nodes** and **blood vessels** surrounding the rectum will

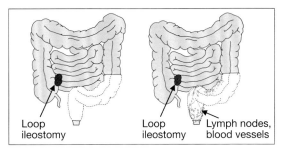

Loop ileostomy   Loop ileostomy   Lymph nodes, blood vessels

also be removed. In both cases the remaining part of your colon and rectum are then joined together. A temporary **loop ileostomy** is usually formed to protect the healing part of intestine.

High anterior resection

This surgery is similar to low anterior resection. However, during a **high anterior resection**, the entire sigmoid colon and only **a small part** of your rectum will be removed. The remaining part of your colon and rectum are then joined together. In rare occasions a temporary **loop ileostomy** is formed to protect the healing part of intestine.

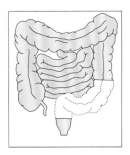

Right hemicolectomy

The right part of your colon will be removed during surgery, while the remainder of your colon will be joined to your small intestine. It is not common for you to have an ileostomy during this operation.

Left hemicolectomy

The left part of your colon will be removed during surgery. The remainder of your colon will be joined together, however, in some cases, your surgeon may decide that the join needs protecting and they will form a temporary loop ileostomy.

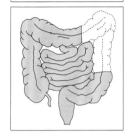

Waking up with an ileostomy

Your ileostomy will usually start working within the first 24 hours after surgery. Immediately after surgery the output would mostly consist of wind (flatus) and a blood-stained liquid called haemoserous fluid. This is completely normal and gradually the blood-stained fluid becomes more greenish/brown in colour and the consistency of the output begins to thicken.

Eventually the output from an ileostomy becomes a semi-liquid (porridge-like) consistency but this depends on how much small intestine was removed during surgery, as well as your dietary routine and food preferences.

Useful advice specific to an ileostomy

- Your ileostomy bag will be **drainable** as your output will always be of a semi-liquid consistency and therefore you would require regular emptying of the bag throughout the day, approximately 5–6 times in 24 hours.
- You will always need to wear a stoma bag as an ileostomy constantly produces output (unless in the shower).
- You may need stoma accessories to help manage the semi-liquid output from an ileostomy. Your stoma nurse will advise on which accessories to use as unnecessary items make your stoma care more complicated and time consuming.
- Change your ileostomy bag every 1–3 days and empty your stoma bag as needed throughout the day. If you are using a two-piece stoma appliance you may change your baseplate every 2–3 days and your stoma bag every day or less often.

Dietary advice

Your ileostomy output may become green and watery when you have not eaten for a few hours or when you first wake up. This is due to an increase in bile production and is completely normal. It should return to normal once you start eating again. People with a new ileostomy may have to be more careful when introducing foods and may need to wait slightly longer to introduce food and fluids from the 📖 'avoid lists' in the main diet section. Unfortunately, there may be some high fibre or irritant foods that may always cause a dietary concern and you may have to limit these foods or avoid them completely, even with an established ileostomy.

Common problems associated with an ileostomy

High output ileostomy – occasionally your ileostomy output may increase in volume and become a more liquid/watery consistency. This can occur at any time after surgery and be caused by changes in diet, lifestyle, periods of increased stress, ill health or by pre-existing medical conditions. When you produce too much ileostomy output, you are at risk of 📖 dehydration because the fluids and salts pass too quickly through your intestine, leading to poor absorption of these vital nutrients and fluids. If your **output is more than 1200–1500 ml in 24 hours** this is referred to as a high output stoma. **Appendix 4 details St Mark's Hospital's guide to managing a high output stoma**. Though a high output stoma may resolve within a couple of days, a prolonged high output stoma requires investigating and treatment.

> 🐘 The signs of a high output ileostomy are emptying your stoma bag more often than usual, producing a watery and green coloured output and possibly leakage from your stoma bag.

If you think you are experiencing a high output from your ileostomy it is important to:

- avoid 📖 dehydration by replacing excessive salt/potassium losses
- include foods rich in potassium – bananas, smooth peanut butter, potatoes, oranges but with no piths and seeds
- avoid intestine irritant foods such as high fibre and spicy foods
- add more salt to your diet or eat salty snacks such as crisps, cheese, crackers and savoury biscuits (without nuts and seeds)
- try not to eat and drink at the same time as this will move food through the intestine more quickly
- eat small regular meals

- include foods that thicken your output
- use medication such as Loperamide (Imodium®) which is available without a prescription or Codeine Phosphate which is only available on prescription
- drink **1 litre a day of isotonic fluids** such as rehydrating drinks, St Mark's E–mix or Dioralyte™
- avoid drinking too much water, **limit hypotonic and hypertonic fluids to 500 ml–1 litre in 24 hours**
- seek medical advice if unsure

> ⚠ If you have tried everything above and your stoma output continues to be high or worsens after 2–3 days, contact your GP or stoma nurse.

Types of fluids		
Isotonic fluids	Hypotonic fluids	Hypertonic fluids
Fluids such as rehydration solutions (Dioralyte™ and St Mark's E–Mix) and drinks rich in salt (vegetable/meat stock, Oxo®, Bovril®, Knorr®) have ideal concentration of salt which helps your body achieve balance and stay hydrated by keeping water and salt in your body rather than moving it to your intestine where it is lost through the stoma.	Fluids such as tea, coffee, 'diet' drinks, water and squash bring salt from your body into your intestine.	Fluids such as juice, alcohol, energy drinks, fizzy drinks and Ensure® drinks bring water together with salt from your body into your intestine.
	Ironically, the more **hypotonic** and **hypertonic** fluids you drink, the thirstier you feel, as once salt and water are brought into your intestine you then start losing them through your stoma.	

Vitamin B$_{12}$ deficiency – our body does not produce vitamin B$_{12}$ but we obtain it from eating animal products, vitamin B$_{12}$ fortified foods or taking supplements. Vitamin B$_{12}$ is absorbed at the end of the small intestine (terminal ileum) and therefore some people with an ileostomy may have difficulty absorbing vitamin B$_{12}$. Your body usually stores enough vitamin B$_{12}$ for several years, so vitamin B$_{12}$ deficiency is not something to worry about immediately, but it is important to be aware of. It is usually sufficient to eat foods rich in vitamin B$_{12}$ such as poultry, meat, eggs, dairy products, seafood and yeast extract (such as Marmite). You need vitamin B$_{12}$ to make red blood cells, for nerve function and for keeping your brain healthy, therefore it is important to correct vitamin B$_{12}$ deficiency as early as possible.

Signs and symptoms of vitamin B_{12} deficiency	
Blurred vision	Nerve problems such as 'pins and needles' or numbness/tingling in your hands, legs and feet
Pale skin	
Irregular heartbeat (palpitations)	Mood changes such as depression, irritability and behaviour changes
Weak muscles	
Shortness of breath	Memory loss
Anaemia (low red blood cells count)	Difficulty concentrating
Feeling faint, lethargic and tired	Loss of appetite

If you require vitamin B_{12} supplements you may be given oral tablets or more commonly a monthly vitamin B_{12} injection. Your GP may also consider a vitamin B_{12} nasal spray or sublingual (dissolves under your tongue) vitamin B_{12} supplements.

> ⚠ Ask your GP to arrange annual blood tests to monitor your vitamin B_{12} levels, especially if you have signs or symptoms of a low vitamin B_{12} and to determine the best method of supplementation.

Kidney stones – you may be at higher than usual risk of developing kidney stones as important electrolytes and salts such as sodium, bicarbonate, calcium and potassium may be lost through your ileostomy. In order to compensate, your kidneys produce more acidic urine which contributes to stone formation. In addition, chronic dehydration may also contribute to kidney stones formation. This is why it is important to stay hydrated as much as possible and replace your electrolytes losses.

You are also at risk of dehydration and stoma obstruction.

Ileostomy and medications

Having an ileostomy may affect how you absorb certain medications particularly if you have had a large amount of intestine removed, experience episodes of vomiting or if you have a more liquid or high output ileostomy. Therefore, medications that used to work well for you may no longer have the same effect after your surgery and you may need a different dose or form of medication.

Medications used to reduce output – sometimes diet and lifestyle changes may not be significant enough for you to reduce your stoma output and regain an acceptable quality of life, therefore you may benefit from using medications such as:

Loperamide Hydrochloride (Imodium®) – which can be bought over the counter or on prescription and is usually the first choice medication recommended to help slow down and reduce your output. The following tips may help you absorb the medication better and make it more effective:

- Take the tablet 30 minutes before each meal.

- Use as little water as possible to swallow the capsules.

- If you find it difficult to swallow the capsules or need many capsules in a dose, try different forms such as sublingual (under the tongue) or suspension (liquid), however, these preparations may be high in sugar and increase your ileostomy output further, especially if high doses and volumes are required. Alternatively, some patients on high dose of Loperamide may benefit from opening the capsules and mixing them with a small amount of water, jam or yogurt.

- Loperamide can be increased safely to doses above 16 mg in 24 hours, however, this should only be done with the recommendation of your stoma nurse or GP. You should always start with the lowest dose possible and increase slowly.

- Titrate the dose of Loperamide to your lifestyle, for example you may need less tablets in the day but more if going out or before bed.

- It may be easier to remember to take Loperamide if you leave some tablets at your bedside and take them as soon as you wake up or before you go to bed.

- If Loperamide does not seem to work after taking it for 2–3 days and trying all of the above tips, contact you GP or stoma nurse as you may have a stomach bug or infection such as Clostridium difficile and Loperamide should not be used.

Codeine Phosphate – is usually prescribed for pain relief but the side effect is constipation, therefore can be used to reduce stoma output. Some patients may prefer using other medications which contain Codeine, such as Co-codamol, Dihydrocodeine, Co-dydramol. Codeine Phosphate can be taken with Loperamide, if Loperamide is not effective on its own but may cause drowsiness, so it is best to take at night. Codeine Phosphate is available only on prescription.

Anti-secretory medications – are useful if the stomach produces too much gastric secretions (digestive enzymes) which can lead to an increased ileostomy output. Medications such as Omeprazole, Lansoprazole and Octreotide are often used to reduce gastric secretions. You usually take these orally except Octreotide which is given as an injection.

Laxatives – are rarely suggested with an ileostomy as they may cause severe fluid and electrolytes losses and 📖 dehydration. It is very unlikely to be 'constipated' with an ileostomy, therefore, if you experience reduced or no output from your ileostomy, you are more likely to be experiencing stoma obstruction.

> ⚠️ If you are required to use laxatives as part of bowel preparation before endoscopy examination or surgery, remind your medical team that you have an ileostomy and it is highly unlikely you will need laxatives.

5. Colostomy

Each year more than 11,000 new patients[2] in the UK undergo colostomy formation. This figure includes patients with either a permanent or temporary colostomy.

On average, a colostomy produces around 300–500 ml per day of semi-formed to solid output and varies from being active up to three times a day to three times a week. A colostomy is usually formed on the left side of your abdomen, though this is not always the case and will depend on your personal circumstances, anatomy and other pre-existing medical conditions. A colostomy may be fashioned as an end, loop or double-barrel stoma.

Types of operations that may require a colostomy

☐ Hartmann's procedure

Part of your large intestine (sigmoid colon) and the upper part of your rectum will be removed during surgery. The diseased colon is removed and the two ends of your colon are not re-joined. An **end colostomy** will be formed. The remaining rectum (rectal stump) will be sewn up and left inside your abdomen. Your rectal stump will continue to produce mucus, which is normal and you may experience a mucus discharge from your anus. Once you are feeling better and your intestine has healed, a second operation may be performed to join the colon and your remaining rectum, though this is not always possible.

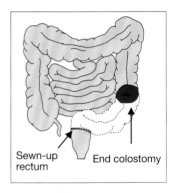

Sewn-up rectum   End colostomy

☐ Sigmoid colectomy

Part of your large intestine (sigmoid colon) and the upper part of your rectum will be removed during surgery. The rectum is then joined to your large intestine. Sometimes it may not be possible to join the two ends of intestine immediately and an **end colostomy** may be formed.

☐ Abdominoperineal Excision of Rectum (APER)

In this operation the sigmoid colon, rectum and anus are removed through the abdomen and the back passage, in a combination of surgical techniques. Your back passage will be closed with stitches during this surgery and a **permanent end colostomy** is formed.

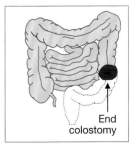

End colostomy

☐ Posterior pelvic exenteration

In women the cervix, ovaries, part or the entire vagina and the uterus (womb) are removed. In case the vagina is removed, you may have a vaginal reconstruction. In men the prostate and seminal vesicles are removed. The rectum and sometimes the anus are also removed. If both your rectum and anus are removed during surgery, your back passage will be closed with stitches. A **permanent end colostomy** is formed.

☐ Total pelvic exenteration

In women the bladder, cervix, ovaries, part or the entire vagina and the uterus (womb) are removed. In case the vagina is removed, you may have a vaginal reconstruction. In men the bladder, prostate and seminal vesicles are removed. Because your bladder is removed a **permanent urostomy** is formed. The rectum and sometimes the anus are also removed. If your rectum and anus are removed during surgery, your back passage will be closed and a **permanent end colostomy** is formed.

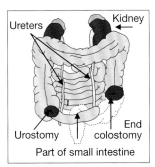

Waking up with a colostomy

Your colostomy will usually start working within the first 2–3 days after surgery. Immediately after surgery the output would mostly consist of wind (flatus) and blood-stained liquid called haemoserous fluid. This is completely normal and gradually the blood-stained fluid becomes more greenish/brown in colour and the consistency thickens. Within a couple of weeks the consistency from a colostomy will be semi-formed or solid output but this depends on how much intestine was removed during the operation, as well as your dietary routine and food preferences. It is not unusual for your stoma nurse to recommend that you use a drainable stoma appliance until your colostomy output is more solid before using closed bags. If you are ready for discharge from hospital and your colostomy output is still quite liquid or not working much, you will be safe to go home as long as you feel well.

Useful advice specific to a colostomy

- Your colostomy bag will be **closed** as your output will usually be semi-formed or solid consistency and therefore you would require changing your bag throughout the day, approximately 1–3 times in 24 hours.
- Some people prefer to use a two-piece system as you only have to change the bag and not the baseplate when you have a bowel motion or can swap between closed and drainable bags easily.

- You may benefit from wearing a drainable bag, if your output is more liquid.

- You **do not** have to empty a closed bag before disposal, however, some people empty the bag by squeezing the output to the top of the bag or cutting the bottom of the bag.

- You may prefer to use a flushable stoma bag for easier disposal but you **must ensure** your stoma bag is flushable before attempting to do so.

- You may be able to take your stoma bag off, for example in the shower, as there will be times in the day the colostomy does not produce output.

- Some people choose to perform colostomy irrigation, which reduces the frequency of bowel movements so you can use a stoma cap/plug instead of a stoma bag.

- Some people can use a stoma cap/plug during activities such as sports, swimming and intimate moments, however, due to their small size these must only be worn for a short period of time and if you are confident of your bowel pattern.

- It is unlikely you will need stoma accessories to help manage the output from a colostomy. Your stoma nurse will advise if you require accessories as unnecessary items make your stoma care more complicated and time consuming.

- Changing your bag depends on the system you use. If you use a:

  - **One-piece drainable** system, change your bag every 1–3 days and **empty** your stoma bag as needed throughout the day.

  - **One-piece closed** system, you may need to change your bag 1–3 times a day.

  - **Two-piece closed** system, you may change your baseplate every 2–3 days and your colostomy bag 1–3 times a day.

Dietary advice

People with a new colostomy can usually reintroduce most foods within a few weeks of surgery but others may need to wait slightly longer to introduce food and fluids from the 📖 'avoid lists' in the main diet section. Most people with an established colostomy can tolerate a normal diet with no dietary restrictions. Your colostomy output may become loose or more liquid if you have not eaten for a few days, if you drink a lot of fluid or if you have overindulged in spicy/irritant foods or alcoholic beverages.

Common problems associated with a colostomy

Constipation – is generally described as having fewer than 3 bowel movements a week. If you change your colostomy bag fewer than 3 times a week and the output is dry/hard or notice a small bulge around the stoma, which disappears once the colostomy works, it is likely you are constipated. Constipation is common with a colostomy, especially if you were experiencing constipation before your operation. To prevent constipation:

- Eat **more** foods rich in fibre such as wholemeal bread/pasta/chapatti, brown rice, vegetables, pulses and fruit

- Eat **less** foods with low fibre content such as white varieties of bread, pasta and rice

- 📖 Refer to **'may increase stoma output'** food chart for useful foods to help manage constipation

- Exercise such as walking is a good way to keep yourself active

- Use laxatives, however, these should be taken on the advice of your stoma nurse or GP

- If you are taking any medication that causes constipation such as some painkillers, consult your GP to consider different medications, if appropriate

- Drink 1.5–2 litres or 8–10 glasses of fluid per day

> ⚠️ If you have been advised to restrict your fluid intake for other medical conditions such as heart problems or kidney problems consult your GP.

Pancaking – sometimes thick, sticky stoma output collects on the top of your stoma rather than dropping down into the bag. This process is called pancaking and can become frustrating if it causes the bag to lift off the skin. Pancaking could also lead to 📖 sore skin as stoma output may sit on your skin. The most common reason for pancaking is lack of air in the bag, creating a vacuum or your output being too thick. To reduce the effects of pancaking:

- **Check your stoma bag filter** – the filter is designed to release air from your stoma bag and at the same time absorb odour. Sometimes the stoma bag filter may work too well and creates a vacuum by removing all the air from the bag. You can try using the little stickers that usually come in the box with your stoma bags to cover some or all of the filter and prevent it from releasing too much air.

- **Let air in** – most modern stoma bags have filters but if your bag does not have a filter, try blowing air inside the bag before applying it.

- **Dietary changes** – if you notice that your output is too thick and sticky, try adding more fibre to your diet and drinking more liquids, **unless you have been advised to restrict fluid intake for other medical** conditions.

- **Stool softener/laxatives** – may be beneficial in the short term. These may be taken orally or via a suppository or enema inserted directly into the colostomy.

- **Use lubricant/oil** – try putting a drop of lubricating jelly, cooking or baby oil **inside** the stoma bag and rub it around before you put the bag on. Make sure you apply lubricant/oil only at the top of the stoma bag and not near the filter or baseplate as this may prevent your bag from sticking to your skin.

- **Try wearing loose clothes** – if you wear tight-fitting clothes, make sure you have enough room for the stoma output to drop into the bag.

- **Use a piece of toilet tissue** – tightly roll up a small piece of toilet tissue into a ball and put it inside the bag. This should prevent the sides of the bag from sticking together.

- **Colostomy irrigation** – may be effective for some people in the management of pancaking.

- **Try a different stoma bag type** – consider using a two-piece or a drainable stoma bag so that you can occasionally open it and allow air to enter inside the bag.

- **Soft convex appliance** – if the above tips do not resolve pancaking, it may be useful considering a soft convex baseplate, which may resolve the associated issues with leakage.

> If you have tried the advice above and are still experiencing problems, contact your stoma nurse for advice.

Diarrhoea – you can occasionally experience episodes of loose stool or diarrhoea with a colostomy from not only dietary changes but the use of antibiotics, chemotherapy treatment or by catching a stomach bug or infection. You are therefore at risk of 📖 dehydration and it is important to treat symptoms of dehydration as soon as possible.

Obstruction – is usually caused by an undigested food (bolus) that obstructs the output flow or by chronic constipation. Sometimes obstructive symptoms in a colostomy may also be caused by 📖 stenosis or 📖 retraction of the stoma itself. Your colostomy obstruction may be **complete** where nothing comes out or **partial**, where some watery output may continue to pass. Either way you should contact your stoma nurse for advice. **Appendix 3 details St Mark's Hospital's guide to management of stoma obstruction.**

Colostomy and medications

Having a colostomy generally does not affect how you absorb medication, however, certain medications may change your stoma output and therefore you should be aware of possible side effects before taking them.

Opioids – may cause nausea, vomiting and constipation, therefore 📖 dehydration may occur.

Laxatives – may be advised as a treatment for constipation or be used for bowel preparation before surgery or endoscopic procedures but may also cause 📖 dehydration.

Colostomy irrigation

Some people have the possibility to achieve a certain level of control over their colostomy function by using a procedure called irrigation, however, they must meet certain criteria (see tables below) and have gained consent from their surgeon. Colostomy irrigation is a procedure whereby water is introduced into the large intestine through your colostomy to help empty the bowel. The water distends your intestine causing wave-like motions (peristalsis) that expel stool and wind (flatus) from your large intestine. It will take time and practice before you achieve good results but unfortunately, even with the best technique, irrigation may not be effective for everyone long term.

If irrigation is right for you, your stoma nurse will book an appointment to see you in clinic, discuss irrigation and teach you how to irrigate your colostomy. This may be done in the hospital or in your home, however, if you are prone to a vasovagal reaction, where you become nauseated, lightheaded or faint, it may be suitable for you to be trained in the hospital setting for the first time. You will be taught and assessed for up to 3 days, then be followed up in a telephone clinic in 1–2 weeks to see how you are coping. You can always contact your stoma nurse if you have any queries or concerns.

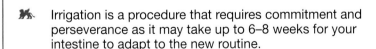

> Irrigation is a procedure that requires commitment and perseverance as it may take up to 6–8 weeks for your intestine to adapt to the new routine.

Advantages of irrigation:

- up to 72 hours without a bowel motion between irrigations (breakthrough)
- allows a level of control over your colostomy
- eliminates or reduces the need of a colostomy bag

- a discreet stoma cap or plug may be used
- reduced odour and wind
- improved body image and confidence
- may reduce anxiety
- may improve constipation
- may help prevent/improve peristomal skin irritation

Disadvantages of irrigation:

- time consuming, it may take up to 60 minutes or more
- it requires uninterrupted periods of time in the toilet
- irrigation must be continued whilst on holiday or abroad
- may have unexpected stoma output between irrigations
- may still need to use colostomy bags
- may have to stop irrigation if your health changes

Inclusion criteria to be considered for irrigation:

Stoma related	Personal circumstances
An end, descending or sigmoid colon colostomy Stoma which regularly produces semi-formed or formed output An established stoma – at least 2–3 months post colostomy formation	Lifestyle that allows you to irrigate Personal commitment and motivation Ability to irrigate on holiday or away from usual facilities Understanding that you may have to wear an appliance of some sort occasionally
Medical assessment	**Environmental**
Written consent from your surgeon	Access to toilet facilities for prolonged periods of time

Exclusion criteria for irrigation:

Intestinal problems	Other comorbidities
Active bowel disease, example diverticular disease, Crohn's disease	Cardiac disease that may cause fluid overload
Irritable bowel syndrome	Renal disease that may cause fluid overload
Fistulae	Cognitive impairment
Persistent diarrhoea	
Existing colon cancer	**Therapy/treatments**
Strictures	Chemotherapy/radiotherapy in progress
	Radiation damage
Stoma problems	**Physical ability**
Symptomatic parastomal hernia	Visual impairment
Stoma prolapse	Poor manual dexterity
Stoma stenosis	Difficulty seeing stoma

Colostomy irrigation equipment

Irrigation equipment is available on a monthly prescription from your GP, however, certain parts, such as the electrical pump, is issued as a once only request. You will also require good toilet facilities with a sink for **water**, a shelf or somewhere to hang your gravity set if required, **wipes** to clean and dry your stoma, and a **rubbish bag** to dispose of your used colostomy bag and **irrigation sleeve**. You may need **lubricating gel** if the cone is not pre-lubricated.

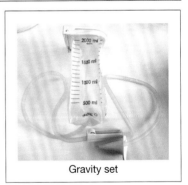
Gravity set

Gravity set – consists of a water container/bag, flexible tubing, a soft cone and a flow-regulating clamp/valve. You need to hang the water container high enough to allow gravity to move the water down the tubing. Some water containers come with an integrated thermometer.

Electric pump set – an electric pump

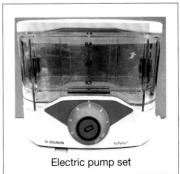
Electric pump set

eliminates the use of gravity when introducing water into your colostomy as the pump pushes the water without the need of gravity. You can adjust the speed of the water flow and monitor the temperature of the water. It comes with its own cones and tubing. However, the disadvantages are that they are more expensive, require additional space compared to a gravity set and require electricity to recharge the battery.

Irrigation sleeve – is attached around your stoma once you remove your used stoma bag. The sleeve allows for the stoma output and water to flow into the toilet bowl. It is single use, therefore you dispose of it once you have completed irrigation.

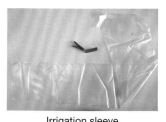

Irrigation sleeve

Stoma plug – is attached to a baseplate and inserted into your stoma in order to stop output from your colostomy. The stoma plug should also allow for wind to pass through an odour-eliminating filter.

Stoma cap – you can wear a stoma cap between irrigations instead of your regular colostomy bag.

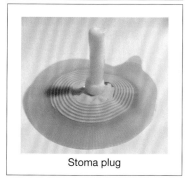

Stoma plug

Appendix 5 details St Mark's Hospital troubleshooting guide for colostomy irrigation.

> ⚠ You should stop irrigating immediately and consult your stoma nurse if you think you have developed a 📖 stoma prolapse, a 📖 parastomal hernia or 📖 stenosis, as these conditions may make irrigation difficult or impossible.

Irrigation – hints and tips

- Plan irrigation during times that you would not be interrupted for at least 60 minutes.
- Try to irrigate at the same time every day, to establish an intestinal routine.
- Try to irrigate your colostomy around the same time you usually opened your bowels before your operation.
- Irrigation may be more effective after a meal or warm drink.

- Do not irrigate if you are ill or experiencing diarrhoea.

- Do not irrigate if you notice a bulge or hernia around your stoma and contact your stoma nurse for advice.

- Avoid becoming dehydrated, as your intestine may absorb the irrigation water resulting in unsuccessful irrigation.

- You may need to irrigate daily at first and gradually extend the time between irrigations once your intestine has adapted.

- Start irrigating with 500 ml of water and gradually increase the volume if tolerated to 750 ml and 1000 ml in the next few irrigations. **Do not** increase water volume beyond 1000 ml without speaking to your stoma nurse.

- The water should always be lukewarm (37°C) as hot water may cause trauma to your stoma and cold water may cause abdominal cramping.

- If your tap water is safe to drink, it is safe to use for irrigation. If you travel abroad and you are unsure if the water is safe for irrigation, **use bottled water**. Make sure bottled water is lukewarm by running the bottle under hot water or immersing it into a bowl of hot water. It is advisable to use a thermometer to check the temperature.

- Wear a small stoma bag rather than a stoma cap during the first 6–8 weeks while your intestine is still adjusting to a routine as your stoma may be active between irrigations.

- It is normal for irrigation to take you longer to complete while you are still learning, however, once you have established a routine, irrigation usually takes approximately 45 minutes to complete.

- It is important to remain determined and committed, even if you experience setbacks.

- If you cannot achieve longer than 24 hours without the colostomy being active, return to daily irrigation or consult your stoma nurse as you may have to increase the water volume or review if the procedure is still suitable for you.

⚠️   Do not attempt irrigation without written consent from your surgeon and without adequate teaching and assessment from your stoma nurse.

Step-by-step colostomy irrigation procedure

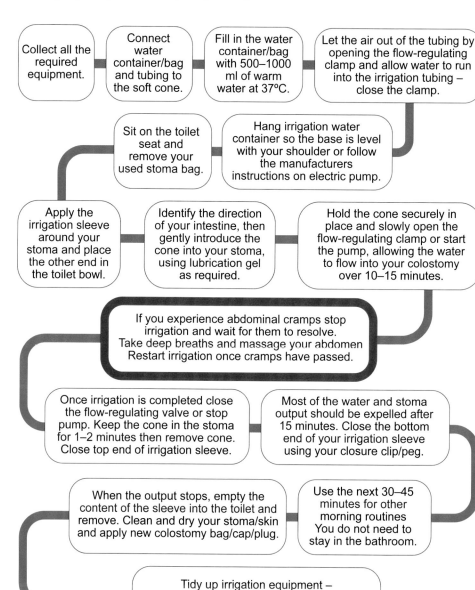

Collect all the required equipment.

Connect water container/bag and tubing to the soft cone.

Fill in the water container/bag with 500–1000 ml of warm water at 37°C.

Let the air out of the tubing by opening the flow-regulating clamp and allow water to run into the irrigation tubing – close the clamp.

Sit on the toilet seat and remove your used stoma bag.

Hang irrigation water container so the base is level with your shoulder or follow the manufacturers instructions on electric pump.

Apply the irrigation sleeve around your stoma and place the other end in the toilet bowl.

Identify the direction of your intestine, then gently introduce the cone into your stoma, using lubrication gel as required.

Hold the cone securely in place and slowly open the flow-regulating clamp or start the pump, allowing the water to flow into your colostomy over 10–15 minutes.

If you experience abdominal cramps stop irrigation and wait for them to resolve.
Take deep breaths and massage your abdomen
Restart irrigation once cramps have passed.

Once irrigation is completed close the flow-regulating valve or stop pump. Keep the cone in the stoma for 1–2 minutes then remove cone. Close top end of irrigation sleeve.

Most of the water and stoma output should be expelled after 15 minutes. Close the bottom end of your irrigation sleeve using your closure clip/peg.

When the output stops, empty the content of the sleeve into the toilet and remove. Clean and dry your stoma/skin and apply new colostomy bag/cap/plug.

Use the next 30–45 minutes for other morning routines You do not need to stay in the bathroom.

Tidy up irrigation equipment – water bag/pump, tubing, stoma cone. Dispose of irrigation sleeve (it is single use only).

6. Urostomy

There are around 11,000 urostomy patients[2] in the UK with over 1,600 new patients[2] each year. A urostomy is a permanent stoma as the bladder is removed during surgery.

'Urostomy' is the general term used for urinary diversion stomas but the most common is the **ileal-conduit**, which is formed using a part of the ileum (small intestine) to carry the urine. On average, a urostomy produces around 1000–2000 ml per day of urine but this depends on your physical size and how much you drink.

A urostomy is usually formed on the right side of your abdomen, though this is not always the case and will depend on your personal circumstances, anatomy and other pre-existing medical conditions. A urostomy is formed as an end stoma.

Types of operations that may require a urostomy

☐ **Cystectomy**

Your bladder will be removed due to underlying disease or trauma. In men the prostate may also be removed. A **permanent urostomy** is formed.

☐ **Anterior pelvic exenteration**

In women the bladder, cervix, ovaries, part or the entire vagina and the uterus (womb) are removed. If the vagina is removed, you may have a vaginal reconstruction. In men the bladder, prostate and seminal vesicles are removed. A **permanent urostomy** is formed.

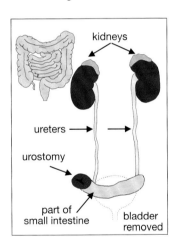

kidneys

ureters

urostomy

part of small intestine

bladder removed

☐ **Total pelvic exenteration**

In women the bladder, cervix, ovaries, part or the entire vagina and the uterus (womb) are removed. In case the vagina is removed, you may have a vaginal reconstruction. In men the bladder, prostate and seminal vesicles are removed. A **permanent urostomy** is formed. The rectum and sometimes the anus are also removed. If your rectum and anus are removed during surgery, your back passage will be closed and a **permanent end colostomy** is formed.

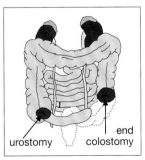

urostomy

end colostomy

Waking up with a urostomy

Your urostomy will start working immediately and will be dribbling blood-stained urine (haematuria) almost constantly. Within a few days your urine will gradually get clearer. A urostomy also produces mucus, as this is the natural lubricant produced by your small intestine, therefore it is normal to have thick, cloudy bits of mucus mixed in with your urine. You will also wake up with two little tubes dangling from your urostomy (stents) which help keep your ureters open while they are healing. Your stoma nurse will show you how to handle the stents **as care must be taken not to pull on the stents while changing your urostomy bag**. If you find it difficult to place the stents into the

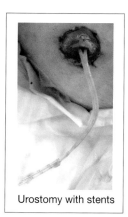

Urostomy with stents

bag it may be useful to use a two-piece appliance while the stents are in place. The stents will be removed in around 10–14 days after your operation but sometimes they may be left in longer and fall out on their own. Mucus may build up and obstruct the stents but if you are able to drink enough water, this will help flush the mucus through and prevent a build-up.

Useful advice specific to a urostomy

- Your stoma bag will be **drainable with a tap**, as your output will always be a liquid consistency and therefore you would require regular emptying of the bag throughout the day approximately 6–8 times in 24 hours.

- Your stoma bag has an anti-reflux valve, preventing your urine from flowing back to your urostomy once in the bag.

- You will always need to wear a bag as a urostomy constantly produces output.

- You may need stoma accessories to help manage the liquid output from a urostomy and protect your skin. Your stoma nurse will advise on which accessories to use as unnecessary items make your stoma care more complicated and time consuming.

- You may also use a **leg bag** in the day which connects to your urostomy bag and collects urine so you avoid having to empty your urostomy bag as often. A leg bag comes in three sizes – 350 ml, 500 ml and 750 ml.

- You can secure the leg bag either with leg straps or a calf sleeve in order to prevent twisting and kinking of the tube. These are available on prescription.

- Change your urostomy bag every 2 days and empty your stoma bag as needed throughout the day. If you are using a two-piece stoma appliance you may change your baseplate every 2–3 days and your stoma bag more often.

- It may help to stop drinking for up to 60 minutes before changing your bag.

- As the urostomy constantly dribbles urine, make sure the skin is completely dry **before** sticking the baseplate.

- Empty your bag before going to bed, but you may also benefit from using a **night drainage bag and a stand**. This is a 2000 ml collection bag and tube, which you can connect to your urostomy bag using an adapter to avoid having to wake up to empty your urostomy bag. Ensure the tubing fits securely to your stoma bag and the tap is turned to the **on** position.

- Always make sure that your night drainage bag is lower than the level of the bed to allow a proper drainage.

- Some manufacturers produce night drainage bags with extended tubing to enable more movement and some night drainage bags have anti-kink tubing.

- Replace the night drainage bag and your adapter (if applicable) once every 7 days.

> 🐾 If you have two stomas – a urostomy and an ileostomy, colostomy or a jejunostomy – you will need to change your urostomy bag first in order to avoid cross-contamination and urinary tract infection.

Dietary advice

Your diet is not affected by having a urostomy, however, caution should be taken with some foods as they can change the colour or the smell of your urine and it can become quite offensive. Refer to the 📖 'diet with a stoma' section on foods that increase/reduce stoma odour and change output colour.

Common problems associated with a urostomy

Urinary tract infection (UTI) – one of the most common complications with a urostomy is developing a UTI. The anatomy of your urinary tract now includes small intestine, therefore urinary infection is likely but preventable.

📖 Stenosis of the urostomy may cause recurrent UTIs. If you have a UTI you may notice your urine has an offensive smell, may be cloudier, darker in colour or even blood-stained. You may also develop a fever, abdominal and back pain. If you have symptoms of UTI, you will need a urine sample taken from your urostomy in order to confirm it and determine which antibiotic is most suitable for you. This is usually done at your GP surgery, however, you may be asked to do this at home.

> ⚠ A urine sample should never be taken from the urine already in the stoma bag.

- **Taking a urine sample at home**

  Equipment – cleaning wipes, warm water, paper towels, rubbish bag and a new stoma bag. Your GP surgery will be able to provide a sterile urine collection container and sterile gauze.

  Procedure:

  1. Use paper towels under the urostomy to protect clothing.
  2. Prepare all equipment, place on a clean surface and avoid unnecessary touching of items.
  3. Remove the used urostomy bag and use wipes and water to clean the urostomy and surrounding skin.
  4. Wash hands before proceeding with collection of urine sample.
  5. Clean urostomy carefully with water, wiping away from the stoma opening, using a circular motion (use new wipe for each wiping motion).
  6. Use sterile gauze to dry the stoma.
  7. Discard the first few drops of urine by letting the urine drip onto the gauze.
  8. Collect urine directly from the urostomy using sterile urine collection container by placing the container under the stoma. Avoid unnecessary touching of the top of the urine container as this may contaminate the sample. Collecting enough urine may take up to 15 minutes.
  9. Dispose of used equipment and wash your hands.

- **Taking a urine sample at your GP surgery or hospital** – if you are unable to collect the sample yourself and need to go to your GP surgery or a hospital, the doctor or nurse may need to insert a small tube (catheter) inside the urostomy in order to collect the urine sample.

- **Prevention of UTI** – in order to avoid frequent urinary tract infections, it is important to keep well hydrated (drink 1.5–2 litres per day, unless advised otherwise). Some people with a urostomy find that by changing the naturally alkaline pH of the urine to a **more acidic pH** the occurrence of UTIs reduces. This can be achieved by drinking 250 ml of cranberry juice twice daily or using cranberry supplement tablets and increasing vitamin C intake. Having a more acidic urine output may also slow down mucus formation.

> A urostomy is made out of a piece of small intestine, therefore a urine sample would usually test positive for intestinal bacteria and should only be treated with antibiotics if you also have associated symptoms of a fever, chills and back pain.

Crystal formation – occurs if the peristomal skin is repeatedly exposed to alkaline urine. These crystals appear as hard white or grey coloured lumps on the stoma itself or the peristomal skin and can cause pain and bleeding. In some cases crystal formation may even cause the urostomy bag to leak which worsens the problem. It is important to protect the peristomal skin and use a well-fitting baseplate. Cleaning the peristomal skin with a 50/50 solution of white vinegar diluted in water seems to be helpful in reducing the crystals as does keeping the pH of the urine more acidic.

Sexual dysfunction – during your operation it is common for the structures involved in reproduction to get damaged. It is therefore important to discuss any sexual concerns with your GP, surgeon or stoma nurse who can refer you to the appropriate team.

Vitamin B$_{12}$ deficiency – may occur as a part of your small intestine (ileum) is removed to form the urostomy. If the end of the small intestine (terminal ileum) is used some people may become deficient in vitamin B$_{12}$ and require supplementation.

Urostomy and medications

Having a urostomy should not interfere with the effectiveness of your medication, however, some medications may change the colour of your urine. Refer to the 'diet with a stoma' section on foods/medications that change output colour.

> ⚠ Warfarin is a medication commonly used to thin the blood. You should not drink cranberry juice if you are on Warfarin, as it increases the effect of Warfarin and your blood may become too thin.

7. Jejunostomy

It is not clear how many people in the UK undergo jejunostomy formation each year because these are not common intestinal stomas. A jejunostomy may be either permanent or temporary.

On average, a jejunostomy produces around 1500–2000 ml per day of a liquid to semi-liquid output, however, it is not uncommon for a normal output to range up to 3000–3500 ml per day. A jejunostomy is a high output stoma and you most likely would require nutritional supplementation in order to prevent complications such as 📖 dehydration, electrolyte imbalance and malnutrition.

A jejunostomy is usually formed on the right side of your abdomen, though this is not always the case and will depend on your personal circumstances, anatomy and other pre-existing medical conditions. A jejunostomy may be formed as an end, loop or double-barrel stoma.

Types of operations that may require a jejunostomy

☐ Bowel resection

Part of your intestine may need to be removed for different reasons such as perforation, narrowing or necrosis. During your operation, the surgeon may need to remove a significant length of your small and/or large intestine and then join the remaining ends.

Depending on your personal circumstances and disease progression, you may need to have a jejunostomy. Sometimes your surgeon may decide that it is best to give you a **temporary loop jejunostomy** or **double-barrel jejunostomy** to protect the healing part of intestine. While, in very rare occasions, you may require a **permanent end jejunostomy** to be formed.

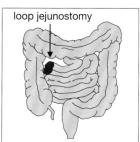
loop jejunostomy

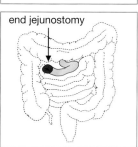
end jejunostomy

Waking up with a jejunostomy

Your jejunostomy will usually start working within the first few hours after surgery producing a blood-stained or greenish/brown liquid.

Eventually the consistency from a jejunostomy may become a semi-liquid consistency but this depends on how much intestine is left behind after surgery as well as your dietary routine and medical restrictions.

Useful advice specific to a jejunostomy

- Your jejunostomy bag will be a **drainable, high output bag with a tap** or a **drainable maxi bag** as your output will always be of a liquid to semi-liquid consistency and therefore you would require regular emptying of the bag throughout the day approximately 6–8 times in 24 hours.

- You will always need to wear a bag as a jejunostomy constantly produces output.

- It is likely you will need stoma accessories to help manage the high and liquid output from a jejunostomy. Your stoma nurse will advise on which accessories to use as unnecessary items make your stoma care more complicated and time consuming.

- Change your jejunostomy bag every 1–3 days and empty your stoma bag as needed throughout the day. If you are using a two-piece stoma appliance you may change your baseplate every 2–3 days and your stoma bag every 1–3 days.

- It may also help to stop eating and drinking completely for up to 60 minutes before changing your bag if your jejunostomy is particularly active or unpredictable.

- Empty your bag before going to bed but you may benefit from using a night drainage bag and a stand. This is a 2000 ml collection bag, which you can connect to your jejunostomy bag, to avoid having to wake up to empty your jejunostomy bag. Ensure the tubing to the bag fits securely to your high output tap and that the tubing is wide enough for thick output or undigested food to pass.

- Always make sure that your night drainage bag is lower than the level of the bed to allow a proper drainage.

- Replace the night drainage bag every 7 days.

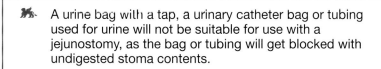

A urine bag with a tap, a urinary catheter bag or tubing used for urine will not be suitable for use with a jejunostomy, as the bag or tubing will get blocked with undigested stoma contents.

Dietary advice

Your jejunostomy output may become green and watery when you have not eaten for a few hours or when you first wake up. This is due to an increase in bile production and is completely normal. It should return to normal once you start eating again. People with a new jejunostomy may have to be more careful when introducing foods and may need to wait slightly longer to introduce foods and fluids from the 📖 'avoid lists' in the main diet section. Unfortunately, there may be some high fibre or irritant foods that may always cause a dietary concern and you may have to limit these foods or avoid them completely, even with an established jejunostomy.

The amount of food and fluid that is absorbed by your jejunum will depend on the length of remaining intestine you have. It is very important with a jejunostomy to chew all food well as food moves quickly through a jejunostomy and undigested food may easily cause a 📖 stoma obstruction. It may be better to eat small, high calorie meals throughout the day and snacks, rather than big meals. It is advisable to add extra salt to your meals. It may also be helpful if you do not eat and drink at the same time and allow 30–60 minutes between eating and drinking. Some people add high-calorie and high-protein drinks and powders to meals. However, avoid drinks high in sugar or artificial sugars as these may increase your stoma output.

Common problems associated with a jejunostomy

Nutritional and electrolytes deficiency

Many people with a jejunostomy usually require nutritional and fluid supplementation as unfortunately there is not enough intestine left to absorb all the water, nutrients and electrolytes you need to maintain your weight and health. The shorter the length of intestine remaining after surgery, the more likely it is that you would need to alter the way you receive nutrition. Some important electrolytes, minerals and vitamins such as magnesium, vitamin B_{12}, vitamin D and sodium may need to be replaced as deficiency is common in jejunostomy patients. This can be done by:

- adding supplements to your oral diet
- using enteral feeds via a nasal gastric tube directly into your stomach or small intestine
- having intravenous fluids with added electrolytes
- receiving intravenous nutritional support (parenteral nutrition)

Supplements and feeds – if you are not absorbing enough nutrients, you may need to be assessed by a dietitian or nutrition nurse to decide what oral supplements and/or enteral feeds you may need added to your diet.

Fluid restriction – you may also have to alter the way you drink fluids. If you have less than **200 cm** of your jejunum remaining after surgery, **restrict oral hypotonic fluids** (water, coffee, tea and squash) and **hypertonic fluids** (juice, fizzy drinks, Ensure®) **to less than 1 litre/day**, while **isotonic rehydration solutions** such as St Mark's E–mix and Dioralyte® should be taken instead to replace losses of sodium.

Intravenous nutritional and fluid supplementation – if you have less than **200 cm** of your jejunum remaining after surgery, you may need to have **intravenous fluids and electrolytes, nutritional supplementation (parenteral nutrition) or both** through your vein in order to compensate the losses of fluids, electrolytes, minerals, vitamins and other vital nutrients.

Nutritional supplementation is given to you as **parenteral nutrition** in a vein overnight, on daily basis or a few times a week. The frequency will depend on your individual nutritional status. Parenteral nutrition may help to decrease the volume of output from your stoma.

Distal limb feeding – involves putting either a nutritional supplement (feed) or reinserting the output from your jejunostomy (chyme) back into your stoma. This is used with some patients to ensure the intestine receives nutrients. You may be considered for distal limb feeding if you have a loop or double-barrel jejunostomy.

Research shows that distal limb feeding may reduce your stoma output and reduce/eliminate the need for fluid and/or nutritional supplementation. Your team of doctors, dietitians and nutrition and stoma nurses will explain everything you need to know about distal limb feeding and teach you the technique.

You are also at risk of the following conditions which are explained further in the 📖 'complications' and 'ileostomy' sections in this book:

- dehydration
- stoma obstruction
- high output stoma
- kidney stones
- vitamin B$_{12}$ deficiency

> It is important to have your bloods (including magnesium, vitamin levels and electrolytes) and urine sodium regularly checked by your GP to prevent or treat possible complications associated with a high jejunostomy output.

Jejunostomy and medications

Medication use is similar to medications with an ileostomy and is explained further in the 'ileostomy' section in this book. However, people with a jejunostomy are even less likely to absorb oral medications because of the insufficient length of remaining intestine, therefore, you may have to take certain medications through your vein, by intramuscular injections or other non-oral forms of medications.

8. Living with a stoma

Travelling

Having a stoma does not mean that you will not be able to travel anymore but you will need to make some adjustments in order to enjoy travelling post-surgery.

It is best to travel once you are confident with managing the stoma and you have settled into a daily routine. When planning to travel the list below will assist in helping plan a stress-free journey.

Travelling checklist:

- [ ] telephone/email of stoma delivery company
- [ ] travel insurance policy
- [ ] stoma travel certificate
- [ ] change of clothing/underwear
- [ ] anti-diarrhoeal medications and rehydration solution
- [ ] RADAR key and/or 'can't wait' card
- [ ] telephone/email of destination stoma nurse/hospital
- [ ] pack double the amount of stoma supplies
- [ ] pre-cut a couple of stoma bags
- [ ] spare products for emergency bag change
- [ ] reserve your seat next to an aisle and near a toilet

Telephone/email of stoma delivery company – before travelling, you may consider obtaining a telephone number or email address of your stoma delivery company in case you run out of supplies and need an urgent supply while away. Many manufacturers offer free shipping of supplies to select countries in case of an emergency, however, it may take a few days before they can send you products, depending where you are. Always remember to take a note of your stoma products type, name, size, item code and manufacturer, as this will ensure the correct products are sent or be helpful in finding a suitable alternative.

Cost of supplies abroad – if you need to obtain stoma supplies abroad, you will need to pay for them. Keep the receipt, as this will help you claim an expenses refund from your travel insurance company, if applicable on your insurance policy.

Telephone/email of destination local stoma nurse – if possible obtain a telephone number or email address of a local stoma nurse or general hospital at the destination you are travelling to in case of an emergency. Make sure you have contact details of your local stoma nurse as well, in case you need assistance with anything.

Buy travel insurance – it is important to buy the correct level of travel insurance for your trip as not all insurance companies cover pre-existing conditions. If your cover is insufficient, any stoma related costs during your travel may not be reimbursed by your insurance policy, therefore make sure your insurance covers stoma related costs. If you have trouble finding the right insurance, contact any of the stoma associations or support groups and ask for up to date travel insurance advice.

Travel certificate – get a travel certificate from your stoma nurse, GP or stoma support association/group and ensure it is stamped and signed. Having a travel certificate is useful as it contains a detailed explanation, in several languages, on what a stoma is, why you need to wear a stoma bag and why you need to keep supplies with you. It may also help if you need to be searched by security, such as in an airport, as this can avoid unnecessary or uncomfortable questioning.

Pack double the stoma supplies – consider the fact that due to weather changes, local food intolerances and other unplanned events, you may need to change your stoma bag more often than you usually do.

- Carry pocket size wet wipes, rubbish bags, pre-cut stoma bags, dry wipes and spare underwear in a small wash bag and keep to hand.
- Take clothes pegs to keep your clothes from getting in the way and to allow your hands to be free to concentrate on your stoma care.
- A small pocket mirror may be useful to check that your stoma is cleaned properly or to secure the bag.

Consider taking drainable bags if you have a colostomy – as well as your usual closed bags, in case the consistency of your output changes.

Consider leg/night bags for a urostomy – to allow more capacity in case you drink more fluids or alcohol and are unable to find toilet facilities.

Reserve your seat next to an aisle and near a toilet – as you will be able to access the toilet easier without disturbing others.

Take anti-diarrhoeal medications and rehydration solution – when travelling to foreign countries hot weather and excessive sweating may cause 📖 dehydration. You may also have some problems with local food intolerances or dietary changes. This is why it is important to take anti-diarrhoeal medications and rehydration solutions in order to be able to manage a 📖 high output stoma, replace electrolytes losses and prevent 📖 dehydration.

Drink bottled water – it is advised to only drink bottled water or cooled, boiled water unless you are certain the drinking water is safe.

Avoid street food – you can still enjoy local cuisine, however, choose recommended establishments to avoid food poisoning and abdominal discomfort or 📖 high output stoma. Be cautious of what ingredients are used so you can isolate problematic foods.

RADAR key or National Key Scheme – is a universal key, which unlocks every accessible toilet in the UK. Some people find it easier changing their stoma bag in an accessible toilet, since there is more space, a wash basin and shelving to place equipment. A RADAR key is usually obtained for a small fee, around £5. Your stoma nurse, support group/association or your GP can provide information on purchasing a RADAR key, however, most stoma delivery companies can provide a key free of charge.

'Can't Wait' card – is a wallet sized, plastic card, which allows you to use a public toilet without having to wait in line. Some shops may even allow you access to staff toilets. The card can be obtained from the stoma support groups/associations as well as many stoma products manufacturers and your stoma nurse.

Sunflower Lanyard – the hidden disabilities Sunflower Lanyard Scheme® is a movement bringing awareness about invisible disabilities with trained personnel on hand to offer help if required. The scheme is currently recognised in the UK, at most airports, rail providers, major supermarkets, NHS Trusts, independent GP surgeries, cinemas, banks and sport venues and is becoming more popular in international airports as well. You can purchase a hidden disabilities Sunflower lanyard from the organisation's website for £1 plus a shipping cost.

Blue Badge Scheme – allows holders of the Blue Badge to use disability parking spots. This right is now extended to hidden disabilities as well. If a stoma patient meets the criteria and scores 10 points under the **Personal Independence Payment (PIP)** mobility test of being "unable to undertake any journey because it would cause overwhelming psychological distress to the claimant" they will be eligible for a Blue Badge.

Hints and tips depending on mode of travel:

Air travel

- Make sure you pack stoma supplies in two separate suitcases using your check-in suitcase and your carry-on suitcase, in case some of your luggage is lost or delayed.
- Remove the stoma appliances from their boxes, as it takes less space, however, be aware it may be easier to store your products in the original packaging once you reach your destination.

- Many airlines allow passengers to carry a small free-of-charge bag with medical equipment, in addition to your carry-on luggage, which in your case will allow you to take your wash bag with stoma care essentials.

- You will not be allowed to carry an adhesive remover spray on the plane, as it is considered flammable. You can ask your stoma nurse to arrange for you to have adhesive remover wipes sent to you instead of sprays as a one-off order.

- You may not be allowed to take scissors in your carry-on luggage, therefore, you will need to pre-cut some stoma bags to keep with you on board. Carry scissors in your checked baggage instead.

- Arrive at the airport early, as you may need extra time to go through security. Remember to have your travel certificate ready and empty your stoma bag before going through security.

- Avoid drinking alcohol or fizzy drinks during your flight as this may make your stoma more erratic or cause the bag to fill with wind.

- Carry bottled water and salty snacks as you can easily get dehydrated on long haul flights.

- Position your seat belt either above or below your stoma.

- Use the toilet before boarding the plane and before meals when it is less busy.

Rail travel

- Not all trains have toilets, so check with the railway company to ensure you are prepared beforehand.

- Use the toilet at the station before you board, as they are more stable than trying to use one on a moving train.

- Some trains do not offer food and drinks services, therefore, consider bringing your own supplies.

Road travel

- Make note of the location of service stations or petrol stations with toilet facilities along your route so you know when you will be able to stop.

- Never leave your stoma supplies in a car in hot weather as the stoma baseplates may melt. It may be a good idea to keep your stoma bags in an insulated bag in hot weather.

- Special attachments are available for your seat belt, which adjust the tension of the belt. You can purchase them from vehicle supplies stores or maternity shops, as these are also used for pregnant women (maternity seat belt adjuster).

- Carry a spare plastic pot with a tight or lockable lid to empty your bag into if you get stuck in traffic and are unable to reach a toilet.

Sea travel

- Toilet facilities on ships and ferries are usually easily accessible, however, if the sea is rough the toilets may be occupied for long periods. Carry your "Can't Wait" card with you to ensure quick access to a toilet.
- Familiarise yourself with the location of toilets as the nearest may be on a different deck.

Clothing

There is no reason for you to change the way you used to dress before your stoma operation, however some people feel more comfortable wearing loose clothing, patterned clothing, longer tops, scarfs, wraps or layered clothes to make the stoma bag less visible and to feel more confident. Low or high-waisted jeans are usually comfortable to wear with a stoma. If you usually wear a belt, you may have to wear it loosely or consider using braces rather than a belt. Some people opt for elasticated waistbands. A belt should not rub across a stoma as it may cause the stoma to bleed. Though you are conscious of your stoma, most people would not know you have a stoma, unless you tell them. Stoma bags are designed to be discreet and not visible through most clothing. It is important to wear the correct size bag as a mini bag though discreet, will be more visible once it begins to fill, than a midi or maxi bag. Also remember to empty/change the bag when it is approximately half-full, as an empty bag is less visible under clothing.

Alternatively, there are quite a few stoma-clothing companies, which produce special underwear, swimwear and high-waisted tights and trousers, though these can usually be purchased from high street shops or online, at a cheaper cost. Underwear and clothing is not usually permitted on prescription.

Returning to work

Returning to work after stoma surgery will usually depend on the type of surgery you have, what type of work you do and the opinion of your surgeon. Usually you should be able to return to work within 6–8 weeks after discharge from hospital but you should consider discussing your options with your employer as soon as possible. You do not need to let your colleagues know that you have a stoma but it may be helpful if your manager is aware so the appropriate measures are put in place, should you need assistance on your return to work. Having a stoma should not prevent you from doing your job, though it may take some time to get your stoma used to your working routine.

To make the transition back to work as smooth as possible:

- Get used to your work routine by waking up at the time you would usually get ready for work and plan your day as if you were at work.
- Take the route into work to see if you would need to stop and empty/ change your bag.
- Map out toilets on the route.
- Consider if you can work from home or on a part-time basis.
- Speak to your manager or occupational health department and discuss your options as you may be able to have a phased return to work which means you work less hours per day for the first few weeks.
- Initially you may need to be assigned different duties, especially if your job is strenuous. Heavy lifting or strenuous activities may put you at risk of developing a 📖 parastomal hernia so you should avoid any heavy lifting for at least 8–12 weeks after surgery.
- If your work involves activities which may cause possible accidental injury to your stoma, you should consider using a **stoma shield** which your stoma nurse can advise on.
- Consider keeping extra stoma supplies and a pair of underwear or a change of clothes at work, in case the stoma bag leaks.

Returning to school

Most schools will allow you to take time to recover from your operation as you would have discussed your plans to continue your education before considering surgery. However, if your operation was an emergency, it is an idea to discuss your options as soon as you feel well enough to do so. To make the transition back to school as smooth as possible:

- Get used to your school routine by waking up at the time you would usually get ready for school and plan your day according to your timetable.
- Take the route into school to see if you would need to stop and empty/ change your bag.
- Map out toilets on the route.
- Give yourself realistic goals and expectations and do not put too much pressure on yourself to catch up with work.
- Discuss with your Head of Year if you feel you need to review your situation at any time.
- If you are struggling to prepare for exams, you could ask for a letter from your surgeon outlying your surgery and possible implications so your school can consider exceptions for you or guide you to a more suitable pathway.

- For younger children, a school nurse may be able to assist with initial problems caused by the stoma or offer support if required.
- If you play contact sports you should consider using a **stoma shield**, which your stoma nurse can advise on.
- Consider keeping extra stoma supplies and a pair of underwear or a change of clothes in your locker, in case the stoma bag leaks.

Driving

You should not drive a vehicle while you are still recovering from your surgery. In your follow-up appointment with the surgeon, at approximately 6–8 weeks post-surgery, they will advise if you are fit enough to drive.

- Always consult your car insurance company, since insurance policies vary in the time recommended for you to resume driving after abdominal surgery. It usually takes at least 6 weeks before it is safe for you to start driving.
- You will need to be able to use the emergency break, reverse and be able to stop suddenly, without being in pain, therefore, it is very important to not only rely on time frames set by your surgeon and insurance company, but listen to your body and only resume driving when you feel emotionally and physically ready to do so.
- You are **not exempt** from wearing a seat belt with a stoma. If your seat belt is putting too much pressure on your abdomen or stoma, you should consider purchasing a **seat belt adjuster** to help make a seat belt more comfortable. You can buy these in car accessories stores and maternity stores, as these are also used by pregnant women (maternity belt adjuster).

Living with children

Depending on the age of your children, it may take time to learn what works best when interacting with them so they understand your new routine and any precautions you may have to take.

- Refrain from lifting children or carrying them around, especially for the first 8–12 weeks after your surgery, as this may contribute to you developing a 📖 parastomal hernia. It may be easier to sit on the floor with them or get older children to climb up to you or ask someone to lift them onto your lap. You may consider using a support garment or support belt when carrying younger children.
- Small children are curious and may try to pull on your stoma bag. It is a good idea to talk to children about your stoma to help them understand and to accept it as part of you, but only if you feel comfortable doing so.

- Some people find it helpful to involve children when changing the stoma bag but this may not be suitable for everyone.
- If you decide to talk to children about your stoma, a helpful approach could be 📖 obtaining a Buttony bear or to make your own toy with a stoma. Colostomy UK also provides a free children's colouring book which explains what a stoma is and why you have one.
- If you are finding it difficult to explain to your child about your stoma you may wish to speak to your stoma nurse or a member of paediatric stoma support groups.
- You should consider using a **stoma shield** if you are concerned that small children may accidentally bump into your stoma while playing.
- Keep your stoma supplies stored away from the reach of small children.

Living with pets

You may have to take some extra precautions when it comes to interacting with pets.

- Avoid lifting and carrying around any pets heavier than 2.5 kg for the first 8–12 weeks after your surgery. Most adult cats and dogs are too heavy for you to lift initially. Even smaller pets such as rabbits and guinea pigs may be difficult to manage, if they move suddenly or kick.
- Be careful when carrying your pet's food and bedding.
- Take extra care when moving or cleaning cages/pens.
- Large animals, such as dogs, goats, sheep and horses may accidentally bump your stoma while running and playing. This does not mean you should not interact with these animals, however, you should consider using a stoma shield during these interactions.
- Be especially careful when playing with cats as they sometimes express their affection by kneading with their paws and may risk piercing your stoma bag with their claws.
- Keep your stoma supplies away from pets, as these can be harmful if ingested.

Exercise and sports

Physical activity is an important part of your rehabilitation after surgery. In fact, the sooner you start mobilising, the speedier your recovery is likely to be. You are encouraged to start mobilising and building up your stamina and endurance from day one following surgery. Having a stoma should not limit your involvement in exercise and sports, as most people return to some form of activity within 6 weeks following surgery. However, it will take time to regain the exercise regime you used to have before your surgery and for some people, a different form of exercise may be more suitable.

- Make sure you empty your stoma bag before engaging in exercise.
- Light exercise, such as walking and gradually increasing the time and distance is a great way to get back to activities in the first few days of returning home.
- Try going up and down the stairs to regain leg strength.
- When exercising away from home, take spare stoma supplies in case the stoma bag leaks. If leakage is a concern when exercising, contact your stoma nurse as you may need a different stoma bag or accessory products.
- Some people find it more reassuring to use flange extenders around their stoma bags to improve their confidence when returning to exercise. Support garments and belts are also useful for adding extra support to the abdomen and stoma appliance during exercise. Your stoma nurse will be able to advise you on different accessory products.
- Avoid straining and lifting heavy weights, especially in the first few weeks after surgery to prevent a 📖 parastomal hernia from developing.
- Keep well hydrated as your body requires extra fluids during physical activities or you risk 📖 dehydration.
- Yoga and Pilates are also suitable for you to stay active though you must still be careful with some positions. Chair yoga is a modified version of yoga, available for people who cannot stand for a prolonged period.
- Once you are able to walk for at least 30 minutes and are confident with your stoma and routine, you may consider sports such as running or cycling.
- Swimming is a great form of exercise and can be relaxing for some people. Stoma appliances are designed to withstand contact with water, however, you may want to change your appliance after swimming to ensure it does not leak. You may consider purchasing stoma swimwear, designed with a special compartment to keep your stoma bag supported when swimming. Some people find multi-coloured/patterned swimsuits or high-waisted shorts more discreet when swimming and can be purchased from a high street shop or online.
- If going to the gym is your preferred method for exercise, it is advisable that you refrain from heavy lifting and start with light exercise for the first 8–12 weeks post-surgery. Gradually build up the intensity as you regain your strength.
- Engaging in contact sports such as football, tennis, rugby, cricket and martial arts should only be started once your body is completely healed

and you feel ready to do so. You may be anxious that your stoma may get bumped but you can wear a **stoma shield**.

Sexuality and body image

Having a stoma may make you feel anxious about your body image or sexuality and many people are overwhelmed about how they look and feel after surgery. Some people worry about how their partner would react to their stoma or how they would start a new relationship, however, with time and emotional support, these concerns are usually resolved. Do not hesitate to talk to your stoma nurse or GP as they are there to offer emotional support and they can speak with you, your partner or family members, if appropriate. Your GP can refer you for more structured psychological support if required.

Body image – you may feel uncomfortable having your stoma bag visible especially when undressing or wearing certain clothes or swimwear. This is a common concern to many people, however:

- Wear clothes that make you feel comfortable and confident as most people will notice how well you look and not the stoma bag.
- Contact support groups or online networks as speaking to other people may help you cope better.
- Use social media to connect with other people with a stoma or view blogs, inspiring pictures, videos and messages.
- Well-being classes, mindfulness, hypnotherapy or complementary and relaxing therapies may be helpful to refocus your thoughts and relieve anxiety, though there is usually a cost associated with these therapies.

Introducing your stoma to others – it is your decision to what extent, if any, you would like your partner, family or friends to be involved with your stoma. Most people have already involved others in their journey towards a stoma and are therefore comfortable with their level of support. If this is not the case or you have a new partner and do not know how to approach the subject, it is important to speak to your stoma nurse as soon as possible. If you are already in a relationship, this may still be a challenging period for both of you and supporting each other is essential.

- Some people find it helpful if their partner is present during initial stoma care teaching in the hospital, so you both can learn how to care for the stoma together.
- You do not have to feel pressured having someone else participate in your stoma care and it is completely your decision who you want to be involved.
- A parent or friend may be equally supportive and in some relationships may be more suitable than your partner. Even if your partner is not actively involved in your stoma care, you can still have a healthy

relationship after surgery.

Sex and intimacy – your stoma should not interfere with you having sex or being intimate with your partner, though it may take some time to rekindle sexual feelings after surgery. There is no set time for when you should be ready to engage with sexual activities as people recover at different times.

- Before engaging in sexual activities make sure that you feel physically and emotionally ready, as your body has undergone major surgery and needs time to recover. Set manageable expectations, as it may take a few months to recover physically and emotionally.

- Initially being intimate without having sexual intercourse is usually sufficient for many couples.

- Communication is very important as your partner may be worried that sexual activity may cause you pain or make you feel pressured and uncomfortable. If sexual intercourse is painful or not possible, you should wait a bit longer before trying again.

- It is not always easy to talk about having a stoma with a potential partner, as people fear negative reactions or rejections. It may be difficult to bring the topic up, but the right person will be able to accept both you and your stoma. You may want to speak to someone who has experienced this situation before and should contact your local stoma support group or association.

Once both you and your partner feel emotionally and physically ready to engage in sexual activity, there are a few tips and hints you may find useful:

- Empty your stoma bag before intimate moments.
- Use a smaller stoma bag or a stoma cap (colostomy only) during sexual activity.
- Buy special stoma underwear with a pocket to hide the bag.
- Wear body suits or high-waisted underwear with poppers or discreet openings.
- Fold the bag and secure it to the abdomen with tape, to prevent movement of the bag.
- Anti-diarrhoeal medication such as Loperamide can be taken before intimate moments to reduce and thicken the stoma output.
- Thickening or gelling sachets can be placed in the stoma bag to reduce the movement of stoma output.

> ⚠   Under no circumstances attempt to use your stoma as part of your sexual activity. Do not introduce anything inside your stoma, as this will most likely become stuck in the stoma or cause damage.

Sexual dysfunction – is usually caused during your operation by damage to the nerves involved in sexual function but may also be a side effect of radiation therapy, advanced disease, surgical technique or level of expertise. Not everyone with a stoma will experience sexual dysfunction, however, if you need an operation that requires the removal of the rectum, bladder, uterus (in women) or prostate (in men), you may be more likely to experience a degree of sexual dysfunction. The most common features in both men and women are loss of libido (the desire to engage in sexual activity), an inability to reach orgasm or psychological concerns such as increased anxiety and reduced body image. These symptoms are usually temporary and resolve within a few months. However, if you are concerned, you should contact your GP, surgeon or stoma nurse, as you may need to be referred to a specialist urologist, gynaecologist or psychologist, who will be able to help you with any prolonged sexual problems.

- **Men** may experience **erectile dysfunction** which is the inability to achieve or maintain an erection. Some men also experience **ejaculatory problems** such as retrograde ejaculation (where sperm enters the bladder instead of the penis, causing you to pass cloudy urine) or you may not ejaculate at all.
- **Women** may experience discomfort and pain during intercourse (dyspareunia), vaginal dryness or loss of sensation.

Fertility, pregnancy and family planning

Fertility or the ability to conceive a baby, in both men and women, may be reduced after stoma surgery commonly due to damage to the prostate or seminal vesicles (in men) or damage to the uterus or scaring around the fallopian tubes (in women). The risk of reduced fertility or the possibility of becoming pregnant depends not only on the degree of damage during surgery or scaring post-operatively but on other factors such as your age, weight, lifestyle, medication use and other medical conditions you may have. The risk of reduced fertility may be increased if chemotherapy or radiation therapy is required as part of your treatment or your operation is performed as an emergency or via open surgery.

Your individual risks must be discussed with your surgeon and GP **before** undergoing surgery. Some people may have the option to start or complete their family before opting for surgery. If this is not the case, fertility preservation methods such as sperm banking, egg harvesting or embryo freezing (of fertilised eggs) may be options to consider, if there is going to be considerable risk to your fertility. Fertility preservation is available free on the NHS if you have cancer and your treatment is NHS funded, but you must also meet all the relevant criteria. You may still have to pay storage fees when your cancer treatment is finished or if you require in-vitro fertilisation (IVF) to get pregnant. You may wish to self-fund for fertility preservation, but you will need to consider the costs of medical consultations, screening tests, freezing charges and ongoing storage expenses.

Pregnancy – a stoma does not prevent you from becoming pregnant though it may take a bit longer and be slightly more challenging both physically and emotionally, especially if you become pregnant quickly after your operation. It is advisable that you wait until you recover fully from surgery, have completed all necessary medical treatments and feel well enough to support a growing baby. People with a stoma usually fall pregnant within 12 months of trying and if this is not the case, speak to your stoma nurse or GP as you or your partner may need to be investigated.

If you become pregnant, you are at a slightly higher risk of stoma complications such as 📖 prolapse or 📖 parastomal hernia due to the increased abdominal pressure as your baby grows. However, the likelihood of you developing a stoma complication also depends on the type of stoma you have, your age, general health, weight and lifestyle. As your pregnancy progresses, you may find it increasingly difficult to see your stoma but a mirror is usually sufficient to assist with bag changes. Occasionally the stoma bag may leak as your abdomen changes shape or the consistency of your stoma output changes but your stoma nurse can assist you with any stoma related concerns.

Family planning – if you are sexually active, you should discuss your birth control options with your family planning (sexual health) clinic as there are many different forms of contraception available. Most people with a stoma do not have problems with contraception, however, women may not absorb oral contraception pills if you have episodes of vomiting or a particularly 📖 high output stoma and may require an alternative method or back-up contraceptive method.

> ⚠️   **Before** undergoing stoma-forming surgery it is important to discuss your risk of sexual dysfunction or reduced fertility, especially in people of childbearing age.

Diagnostic procedures

Occasionally it may be necessary to look inside your stoma with a camera (endoscopy) or X–ray (radiology) to assess the condition of the intestine.

You should always take your stoma equipment with you, as you may have to remove your stoma bag for the procedure and your usual bag may not be available, the stoma output may increase after the procedure, especially if dye was inserted into the intestine or you may have to wait longer than expected in hospital, if you feel unwell after your investigation.

If you are advised to follow a liquid diet or 📖 low fibre/low residue diet before your procedure, it is important to avoid dehydration.

Endoscopic investigations

With a colostomy, you may need to take a bowel-cleansing preparation before the procedure, and you should wear a **drainable** stoma bag as your stoma output will be more liquid and more frequent afterwards. With an ileostomy or jejunostomy you should **not** need to take a bowel-cleansing preparation.

Possible stoma complications after endoscopic investigations:

- Bleeding – especially after a biopsy, which usually resolves on its own.
- Erratic stoma function – it may take a couple of days for your stoma to return to its normal pattern.
- Perforation – of your intestine may occur in rare cases, therefore, seek medical advice if you have prolonged abdominal pain or bleeding from the stoma.

Radiological investigations

Loopogram – is usually performed to assess the health of your kidneys, ureters and small intestine used to create your urostomy (urine stoma). A catheter and contrast dye will be inserted into your stoma and a series of X–rays taken.

Distal contrast study – is used to assess the length of your intestine distal to (below) your stoma, to ensure it is free of disease, obstruction or tears prior to beginning distal limb feeding.

Cultural considerations

The five most represented religions in the UK are Christianity, Hinduism, Judaism, Sikhism and Islam. Each of these religions have different customs, beliefs and expectations regarding people with a stoma.

> ⚠ Some people with a stoma such as the elderly, the very young, pregnant women and those with chronic disease or underlying medical conditions, should seek advice from their GP and religious leaders if they feel their health may be compromised by either fasting or undertaking certain ceremonies or rituals.

Christianity

- There are no restrictions placed on Christians with a stoma.
- Christians observe Lent, which lasts 40 days and some Christians may wish to fast during this period.
- Ash Wednesday and Good Friday are the main fasting days where only one simple meal during the day is permitted, usually without meat.
- Meat is avoided on all Fridays in Lent, but substituting fish is allowed.
- It is important to stay hydrated in order to avoid 📖 dehydration.

Hinduism

- When being marked for a stoma prior to surgery, discuss with your stoma nurse any particular items of clothing that you would need to wear. The sari typically covers the stoma bag and does not cause any discomfort or restrictions. Wearing a dhoti or a kurta should not interfere with the position of a stoma bag.
- Many Hindus prefer a clean, freshly changed stoma bag before praying. Consider asking your stoma nurse to try a two-piece system instead of a one-piece system, as these may be easier for you to manage as you can easily change your stoma bag before prayer.
- More than a third of Hindus are vegetarian, therefore, a diet high in fibre can cause 📖 excessive wind, 📖 stoma obstruction and a 📖 high output stoma.
- Cows are sacred animals, therefore, ask your GP or check the labels on your medication to see if they contain bovine products as alternatives may be available.
- Marshmallows and jelly babies usually contain animal-based gelatine, however, vegan marshmallows are available.
- Fasting is common in Hinduism, though drinking water and having one vegetarian meal a day is usually allowed. It is important to stay hydrated in order to avoid 📖 dehydration.
- Special considerations must be taken during Diwali celebrations, as consumption of too much sugary food may increase your stoma output.
- Hindus may prefer to use running water, rather than a bowl of water to wash their stoma and surrounding skin. You can change your stoma bag in the bathroom, with the tap running. Alternatively, you can shower and remove the bag just before you are about to finish in order to clean your stoma.
- Many Hindus prefer to use their left hand for tasks that are considered unclean, such as stoma care.

Judaism

- There are no restrictions placed on Jewish people with a stoma.
- The Sabbath is observed from sunset on Friday to sunset on Saturday. You should remind nursing staff that if you are discharged from hospital you need to arrive home before the beginning of the Sabbath.
- Jewish people may refuse to change their stoma bag during the Sabbath, therefore, you should plan to change your bag before or after this time.
- Pork, shellfish and any food made from porcine extracts are forbidden, therefore, ask your GP or check the labels on your medication to see if they contain porcine products, as alternatives may be available. Jewish people consider the sanctity of life to be paramount and many may make an exception for certain medications if it is medically necessary.
- Dairy products cannot be prepared with or eaten with meat products. If you need to receive dietary supplements containing dairy products, you can ask for them either before or after a meal.
- Praying with a stoma may cause difficulties due to the positions adopted such as swaying. Ensure your stoma bag is emptied and intact before prayer.
- Ritual immersion mikveh requires being entirely naked and without a stoma bag. However, if faecal output and urine are likely to leak into the water, the stoma bag may be considered as part of your body and allowed to remain on the body.
- Some Jewish people may fast for 24 hours without food and water, therefore, if fasting with a stoma, try to stay hydrated and avoid dehydration.

Sikhism

- Many Sikhs are vegetarian, therefore a diet high in fibre can cause excessive wind, stoma obstruction and a high output stoma.
- Medications containing animal-based gelatine could be replaced with alternative medications.
- Animal products, as long as not consumed, are acceptable to be used. These include medical devices worn on the skin, such as stoma appliances and accessories containing gelatine.
- Marshmallows and jelly babies usually contain animal-based gelatine, however, vegan marshmallows are available.
- Running water is preferred for washing and cleaning, however, a bowl of water can be used for stoma care.
- Being a Sikh, you may not want to have any treatment involving cutting

your hair, including body hair. However, sometimes shaving the skin surrounding your stoma may help your stoma bag stick better.

- Sikhism does not encourage ritual fasting.

Islam

- Some religious rituals and activities may need to be avoided after stoma formation.
- Many Muslims use their left hand for tasks that are considered unclean, such as stoma care.
- Praying with a stoma may cause difficulties due to the positions adopted during prayers such as kneeling and bending. Ensure your stoma bag is emptied and intact before prayer.
- Output from ileostomy or jejunostomy is considered clean, as it is above the umbilicus (belly button). Output from colostomy may be seen as dirty as it is below the umbilicus.
- However, if the stoma is formed above the umbilicus it is not usually seen as dirty. You should discuss this with your stoma nurse **before** your surgery as they may be able to site your stoma above your umbilicus.
- During Ramadan Muslims fast from sunrise to sunset without food or fluids so try to stay hydrated and avoid 📖 dehydration.
- Medications via the nose, mouth or rectal route are not allowed during Ramadan, unless you have the permission of an Imam. Discuss alternative medications with your GP.
- Many Muslim will eat vegetarian diet when away from home, if they are unsure that the meat is Halal. A diet high in fibre can cause 📖 excessive wind, 📖 stoma obstruction and a 📖 high output stoma.

There are legal agreements (fatwas) in Islamic law for people with a stoma, these include the following considerations:

- Faeces are regarded as religiously impure or najees, however, Muslims with a stoma should not be considered najees.
- It is not permitted for people to refuse stoma surgery.
- If it is a surgical option, then a left sided stoma is preferred over the right.
- Muslims with a stoma are classed as madhur (excused) and have the permission to combine prayers so that only three prayers are performed daily instead of five. Wudhu (ritual ablution) must be performed before each prayer. If a stoma is active during prayer, then the person does not have to interrupt prayers and can continue praying as they have no control over this.

- Providing there is no odour and all sensible precautions have been undertaken, Muslims can enter a mosque with a stoma. They are advised, however, to stand towards the end of the row in case the bag leaks.

- Muslims with a stoma should fast during Ramadan if they are able, provided medical advice has been sought. If people with a stoma are unable to fast during summer months, then this can be made up later during shorter fast days during winter months. If long-term condition prevents fasting an option of feeding a poor person/family must be carried out for each day a fast is missed.

- Muslims with a stoma are permitted and advised to perform pilgrimage to Mecca – Hajj. There is no religious restriction to this unless medically contraindicated. Males may wear a t-shirt, rather than traditional plain cotton garments, to conceal the stoma. If this is worn, however, then compensation is required in the form of either a sacrifice, fasting or feeding the poor. A plain stoma belt with little or no stitching is advised as a substitute to a t-shirt.

> If you have any doubts regarding whether or not you can continue to observe your religious beliefs, consult with your religious leader for further advice.

9. Cost of stoma care to the National Health Service (NHS)

> An important role of the stoma nurse is helping you select appropriate and economical, yet high quality stoma appliances and accessories that allow you to return to the lifestyle you desire.

While it is important for you to receive the best care and products for your newly formed stoma, it is also important to understand the growing cost of stoma care to the NHS. Unfortunately, waste caused by the prescribing of unsuitable or unnecessary products has been highlighted as a growing concern.

The NHS covers the majority of the costs related to your essential stoma appliances and accessories, including the related fees associated with the procurement, prescribing, dispensing, customising (cutting the bags to a specific size) and delivering of your stoma products. Some patients are required to pay for a part of their prescription, but a high proportion of patients are exempt from all charges due to their medical or social situation.

The NHS was set up to provide high quality, accessible care for all patients and is funded by the taxes we pay, therefore, remains free at the point of contact, however, even if you are not required to pay for stoma services and products, it is not acceptable to waste them. Rising costs in stoma care is often because of a lack of information and awareness from some stoma products manufacturers, patients, GPs and stoma nurses.

Every week in the UK, thousands of pounds of stoma products are returned to stoma care departments or disposed of in landfills. Unfortunately, we are unable to re-use prescribed stoma products in the UK but luckily some of the unwanted products are shipped by charitable organisations to countries, who cannot afford these products.

In order for the NHS to stay true to its aim, we need to embrace new ways of working without compromising the care stoma patients receive. This can only be achieved if we all do our bit to reduce the inappropriate prescribing of stoma products, prevent waste and prolong the available resources for both current and future patients.

Below is a list of the estimate costs to the NHS for some of the most commonly prescribed products:

Average cost of stoma products		
One-piece system (per item)	**Two-piece system (per item)**	
Ileostomy flat bag £3.10	Ileostomy bag £1.60	
Ileostomy convex bag £4.40	Colostomy bag £1.50	
Colostomy flat bag £2.90	Urostomy bag £3.20	
Colostomy convex bag £3.20	High output bag £3.70	
Urostomy flat bag £5.40	Convex baseplate £4.10	
Urostomy convex bag £5.90	Flat baseplate £3.80	
High output flat bag £3.40		
High output convex bag £4.50		
Accessories		
Barrier wipes (30pc) £22.00 Barrier spray £10.50	Adhesive remover spray £8.00	Barrier rings (1pc) £2.00
	Adhesive remover wipes (30pc) £14.00	Flange extender (20pc) £12.70
		Stoma paste £6.00

Hints and tips to help you monitor the increasing costs of stoma products

Sometimes we only need to make subtle changes in order to help monitor the NHS stoma care spend. You will never be expected to manage without essential stoma care items, however, there are items that are not intended for routine use or can be purchased for a fraction of the cost.

If you are not certain about any of the suggestions below please contact your stoma nurse or GP for clarity, as your local NHS region may have its own prescribing formulary or recommendations.

- **Contact your stoma nurse if you are changing your stoma appliance more frequently, having multiple leakages or using more accessory products than usual** – your stoma nurse can assist you resolve any issues which may have caused you to use more appliances or accessories. If it is necessary to increase your supplies they will contact your GP, stoma delivery company or prescribing hub to authorise the changes so you do not run out of supplies.

- **Contact your stoma nurse if you want to sample a new product** – there are numerous ways to make you aware of new or alternative stoma products, however, with such variety it is easy to become overwhelmed. Your stoma nurse will be able to decide if the product is suitable for your type of stoma and lifestyle before it is added to your prescription. Unsuitable products may actually cause more problems or make stoma care more complex.

- **Do not add new products to your prescription before speaking to a stoma nurse** – all new products need to be authorised by your stoma nurse and GP, however, most GPs do not fully understand which products are most suitable for you and therefore may prescribe the incorrect product or quantity.

- **If you are using less stoma bags than prescribed or if you no longer require an item** – consider reducing your monthly prescription request. Inform your GP, pharmacist, stoma delivery company or prescribing hub when they contact you to re-order and they can change the quantity of products that you receive each month. These products are not removed from your prescription, instead they will only be dispensed when you say you need them. They can also be easily reinstated monthly if your situation changes and you need them more often.

- **Use your adhesive remover spray sparingly** – you do not need an excessive amount of spray when changing your appliance. The correct technique is to gently press the nozzle to release a short burst of liquid between the stoma bag and your skin and wait for a few seconds before easing the bag off the skin. Ideally, with the right technique you only need 3–4 presses of the spray to remove your appliance and on average 2–3 cans of spray per month.

- **Choose either adhesive remover spray or wipes** – do not include both wipes and spray to your regular prescription, as this is usually not necessary. Sprays are more economical than wipes.

- **Measure and cut your stoma baseplate correctly** – if the baseplate opening is cut too large, skin damage will occur and therefore the stoma bags will no longer be suitable for your use.

- **Use of skin protective barrier sprays/wipes** – these products are not intended to be used if your peristomal skin is healthy.

- **Use of stoma protective rings/seals and stoma paste** – your stoma nurse may suggest you trial these products to help resolve ongoing issues with your stoma care. Only when your stoma nurse is certain that the best products are selected should they be added to your prescription.

- **Use of flange extenders/security frames** – in some cases, such as people with a 📖 parastomal hernia, flange extenders/security frames are an essential part of stoma care. However, they should not be used to prolong the life of a leaking stoma appliance or for reassurance that the bag will not leak, unless discussed and agreed by your stoma nurse. Changing to a different bag may be more cost effective.

- **Do not request skin cleansers on prescription** – you do not need special skin cleansers to clean your skin and stoma as warm water and dry wipes are sufficient.

- **Do not request air freshener or odour eliminators on prescription** – you do not require special stoma deodorants to reduce odour when emptying your stoma bag unless instructed by your stoma nurse. You can purchase a pocket-sized air freshener from the supermarket which works just as well.

- **Odour neutralising drops are not essential for your stoma care** – you do need odour neutralising drops as your stoma bag does not release odour. If you notice odour, it is best to check on your appliance for leakage or a blocked filter. If you are worried about odour, contact your stoma nurse.

- **Do not use solidifying sachets unless advised by your stoma nurse** you should not regularly require solidifying agents to thicken your stoma output if you have a balanced diet. Occasionally, solidifying agents may mask stoma problems such as 📖 high output, therefore, these products should only be prescribed if advised by your stoma nurse.

- **Underwear and clothing** – should not be added to your stoma prescription as these can be purchased for a fraction of the cost.

The following two tables are a recommendation of the number of stoma bags and adhesive removers which are prescribed on a monthly basis. However, this may vary according to your local prescribing guidelines.

Stoma accessories average use	
Adhesive remover spray	1–2 cans per box of 30 bags
Adhesive remover wipes	1 wipe per stoma bag
Other stoma accessories may be required, however, your stoma nurse will assess you before these are prescribed.	

Stoma appliances average use		
Type of stoma appliance	Change frequency	Monthly average
Colostomy		
One-piece closed bag	1–3 times a day	30–90 stoma bags
Two-piece closed system	Baseplate every 2–3 days	10–15 baseplates
	Stoma bag 1–3 times a day	30–90 stoma bags
One-piece drainable bag	Every 1–3 days	10–30 stoma bags
Two-piece drainable system	Baseplate every 2–3 days	10–15 baseplates
	Stoma bag every 1–3 days	10–30 stoma bags
Ileostomy		
One-piece drainable bag	Every 1–3 days	10–30 stoma bags
Two-piece drainable system	Baseplate every 2–3 days	10–15 baseplates
	Stoma bag every 1–3 days	10–30 stoma bags
Urostomy		
One-piece urostomy bag	Every 2–3 days	10–20 stoma bags
Two-piece urostomy system	Baseplate and stoma bag every 2–3 days	15 baseplates
		10–20 stoma bags
Urine night drainage bag	Every 7 days	4 bags/month (1 box of 10/every 2 months)
Jejunostomy		
One-piece drainable bag	Every 1–3 days	10–30 stoma bags
Two-piece drainable system	Baseplate every 2–3 days	10–15 baseplates
	Stoma bag every 1–3 days	10–30 stoma bags
Night drainage bag	Every 7 days	4 bags/month (1 box of 10/every 2 months)

10. Psychological support

Having a stoma is overwhelming for many people and it may be emotionally challenging in the first few weeks being at home without the support of your stoma nurse and medical team. It can be very confusing and lonely at times and some people may even begin to feel resentment towards their stoma. It is very important to seek help if you find yourself in a situation where you think you are not coping. There are many ways to get the correct level of support you need to help you accept your stoma and the challenges that come with it.

Nursing and healthcare professional support

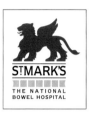

Stoma nurse – your stoma nurse will be there to support you before, during and after stoma-forming surgery. Your local stoma nurses will be able to answer all your questions and offer you both physical and emotional support, however, if for some reason you feel you would like a second opinion, you can always contact the stoma nurses at St Mark's Hospital or another local hospital.

St Mark's Hospital Stoma and Pouch Care Department is a team of specialist nurses with experience in stoma, ileoanal pouch and intestinal fistulae. We are dedicated to providing individualised, expert and research-based nursing care within the field of colorectal surgery. We aim to offer sustainable services for both inpatients and outpatients, providing an exceptional experience for all.

Website: www.stmarkshospital.nhs.uk/stoma-care

Tel: 0208 453 2196, Email: LNWH–tr.stomacare@nhs.net

St Mark's Hospital Inflammatory Bowel Disease Department is a team of specialist nurses offering care to patients with inflammatory bowel disease; providing nursing support, medical treatments, psychological and nutritional support, as well as participating in research and education.

Website: www.stmarkshospital.nhs.uk/inflammatory-bowel-disease

Tel: 0208 453 2368, Email: LNWH–tr.IBDnurse@nhs.net

St Mark's Hospital Polyposis Registry is run by a team of specialists consisting of colorectal surgeons, gastroenterologists, nurse practitioners, nurse specialists and administrators. The team works together to ensure prompt diagnosis and surveillance of patients with or at risk of a Polyposis syndrome. The Polyposis registry team looks after people with a polyposis syndrome and their relatives throughout the patient journey.

Website: www.polyposisregistry.org.uk

Tel: 0208 235 4270, Email: LNWH–tr.polyposisregistry@nhs.net

St Mark's Hospital Psychological Medicine Unit – is dedicated to patients with gastrointestinal disease. The unit offers psychological assessment and support for patients treated at St Mark's Hospital and throughout the UK.

Website: www.stmarkshospital.nhs.uk/services-a-z/psychological-medicine

Telephone aftercare – many stoma delivery and manufacturing companies provide support for stoma patients in the form of telephone services. This is a free service for stoma patients and their immediate family and is usually provided by trained telephone advisors. The advisors are known to the stoma nurses and if they feel you need more support or are concerned with a change in your medical condition, they will refer you back to your stoma nurse. You are not required to use the company's products in order to be considered for their telephone aftercare service, however, you will need to register and sign a consent form to share your personal details. Your stoma nurse will provide all the information about telephone aftercare and arrange for your telephone support to start as early as you would like following discharge from hospital.

Support groups, charities and stoma associations

There are many support groups, charities and associations which offer specific advice and support based on the type of stoma you have. You can meet other people who have experienced life with a stoma or access online information freely but you may have to pay a small membership fee in order to access journals, magazines and to attend information days. Having access to others who have experience with a stoma is usually very helpful as they can share their life experience with you, provide hints and tips on how to manage a stoma on a daily basis and may even share similar hobbies or skills, giving you the reassurance you need to reclaim your life with a stoma. These groups can also offer support to your family, friends or carers.

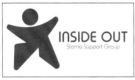

Inside Out Stoma Support Group supports anyone with a stoma and is based at St Mark's Hospital. Website: www.iossg.org.uk Tel: 0208 428 4242 Email: info@iossg.org.uk

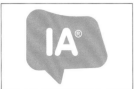

The Ileostomy and Internal Pouch Association (IA) is a registered charity, supporting people living with an ileostomy or internal pouch.

Website: www.iasupport.org Tel: 0800 018 4724 01702 549859, Email: info@iasupport.org

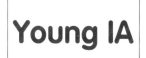

Young IA offers support to young members under the age of 40, either pre-surgery or post-surgery, who undergo either an ileostomy or an internal pouch operation.

Website: young.iasupport.org Tel: 0800 0184 724 / 01702 549859 Email: youngia@iasupport.org

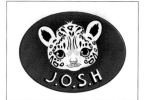

Colostomy UK is a registered charity, supporting people living with a colostomy.

Website: www.colostomyuk.org 24h helpline: 0800 328 4257, Email: info@colostomyuk.org

Junior Ostomy Support Helpline (JOSH) provides support for parents and carers of young people living with a stoma and other bowel and bladder dysfunctions through Colostomy UK.

Website: www.colostomyuk.org/josh
24 hour helpline: 0800 328 4257
Email: info@colostomyuk.org

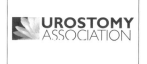

The Urostomy Association is a registered charity, supporting people living with a urostomy.

Website: www.urostomyassociation.org.uk
Tel: 01386 430140
Email: info@urostomyassociation.org.uk

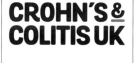

Crohn's & Colitis UK is a charity dedicated to Crohn's disease, Ulcerative Colitis and other forms of Inflammatory Bowel Disease (IBD).

Website: www.crohnsandcolitis.org.uk Tel: 0300 222 5700, Email: helpline@crohnsandcolitis.org.uk

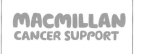

Macmillan Cancer Support Organisation supports patients diagnosed with cancer, offering emotional, physical and financial support, from diagnosis, through their treatment and beyond.

Website: www.macmillan.org.uk Tel: 0808 808 0000

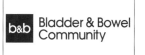

The Bladder & Bowel Community is a support service for people living life with bladder or bowel dysfunction, diversion or condition.

Website: www.bladderandbowel.org
Email: help@bladderandbowel.org

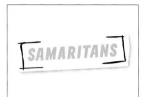

Samaritans is a registered charity aimed at providing emotional support to anyone in emotional distress, struggling to cope or at risk of suicide throughout the United Kingdom and Ireland.

Website: www.samaritans.org
Tel: 116 123, Email: jo@samaritans.org

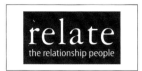

Relate is UK's largest provider of relationship support, regardless of age, backgrounds, sexual orientation or gender identity.

Website: www.relate.org.uk Tel: 0300 0030396

Social media, digital apps and magazines

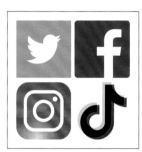

There are also a wide variety of social media communities and lifestyle influencers dedicated to providing physical and psychological support.

You can also search the following hashtag words in order to find some helpful stoma related content on social media: #ostomyawareness #stomaawareness #stoma #ostomy #ileostomy #ileostomybag #ileostomylife #colostomy #colostomybag #colostomylife #urostomy #urostomybag #urostomylife #stomaproud #ostomyproud #stomabag #ostomybag #ostomates #stomalife and #ostomylife.

 Please be mindful with social media content as it may not always be monitored.

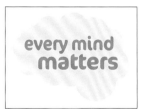

Every Mind Matters provides simple and practical advice to become healthier both physically and mentally. It helps you learn how to deal with stress and anxiety, boost your mood or helps you to sleep better. You can complete an assessment on their website which then provides personalised advice or download free self-help mobile applications.
Website: www.nhs.uk/every-mind-matters

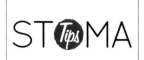

Stoma Tips is a resource for anyone with a stoma containing useful lifestyle tips. Available in paper print and online. You can register and subscribe to receive the magazine through their website.

Website: www.stomatips.com
Email: stomatips@markallengroup.com

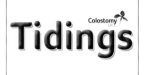

Tidings is a magazine published by Colostomy UK for people with a colostomy. Available in paper print and online. You can download a copy of the magazine from Colostomy UK's website.

Website: www.colostomyuk.org/support/tiding

11. Frequently asked questions

I saw my stoma move, is this normal?

Yes, your intestine constantly contracts and relaxes in a wave-like motion called peristalsis, which is necessary to move the food and fluid along your intestine, through your stoma and into your bag.

You may notice more movement if you use cold water or a cold wipe to clean the stoma or when there is undigested food or constipated stool trying to exit the stoma.

Can I control my stoma output?

You cannot control your bowel or urinary function with a stoma but some people are able to tell when their stoma is going to be active, but they still cannot stop the stoma from working.

Will people know that I have a stoma?

No, not usually, unless you tell them about it. Your stoma bag is designed to be small, discreet and not visible through your clothing.

Can I shower with my stoma?

Yes, you can shower with your stoma either with or without your stoma bag but if you remove your bag, you must have your equipment ready to apply a new bag as soon as you get out the shower. It would also be advisable to choose a time that your stoma is less active.

Is water able to enter my stoma if I take my stoma bag off to shower?

No, peristalsis occurs in one direction – from mouth to anus, therefore, food and fluids do not move backwards or upwards.

Can I have a bath with my stoma?

Yes, you can have a bath with your stoma but you should wait until your abdominal or perianal wounds heal. You must keep your stoma bag on in the bath unless you have a colostomy, irrigate regularly or are confident of when your stoma is active. Relaxing in a warm bath may cause your stoma to become active.

Can I swim with a stoma bag?

Yes, your stoma appliances are designed to withstand contact with water and should not leak. However, empty the stoma bag before swimming and do not swim immediately after meals. You may feel more comfortable wearing specially designed swimwear for people with a stoma.

Do I have to dry my stoma bag after washing or swimming?

Your stoma bag usually has a cover which dries quickly or is waterproof, however, you may prefer to change your bag after washing or swimming.

Why does my stoma change colour?

A healthy stoma is naturally dark pink or red in colour due to the amount of blood supply to the intestine or your general health. If your stoma is pale, grey or black in colour seek immediate medical advice.

Will I feel pain if I touch my stoma?

No, your stoma does not have sensory nerve endings and cannot feel pain but will feel pressure if touched.

Why there is blood when wiping my stoma?

The tiny blood vessels on a stoma can bleed easily when wiped. Spots of blood are normal during cleaning, as long as the blood comes from the surface of the stoma and not from the inside. Occasionally with a new stoma, you may damage a small blood vessel where the stoma is attached to the skin. If this happens apply pressure with a wipe until the bleeding stops.

I see pieces of food in my stoma bag, is this normal?

It is common to see undigested food in your stoma bag but this is less likely if you have a colostomy or chew your food well.

Should I have all my stoma bags pre-cut to my stoma size?

It is not necessary to have your bags pre-cut if you are able to do so yourself, as there is a cost to the NHS for this service. Ideally you should not order pre-cut bags within the first 6 weeks after stoma formation as the stoma will change shape and size, however, it is handy to have a couple of pre-cut bags if you are going out or need to change a bag in an emergency.

What should I do if my stoma bag leaks when I am out?

Always take spare pre-cut stoma bags, adhesive remover spray, wet wipes, dry wipes and a pair of underwear with you so you can change your bag. Some people may carry a sanitary pad, dry wipes or kitchen roll to put around the leaking bag until a toilet can be found.

Where should I empty my stoma bag?

You should empty your stoma bag into a toilet. It may be useful to place toilet paper in the bowl first to stop the stoma output splashing. However, in an emergency, you may be able to empty the contents into a plastic container or plastic rubbish bag, lined with toilet paper to absorb the stoma output, until you are able to find a waste bin.

Where should I change my stoma bag when out?

Preferably use an accessible toilet, as these have more space and facilities, alternatively you can use a regular public toilet. Obtain a RADAR key, which allows you access to every accessible toilet in the UK and a "Can't Wait" card, which allows you to use a public toilet without having to wait.

What should I do if my stoma bag smells when I change it, especially in public toilets?

You can purchase a pocket air freshener/odour neutraliser and use as needed. Remember even people without a stoma may leave a smell after emptying their bowel.

How do I dispose of my soiled equipment once I have changed my stoma bag?

These should be placed in the plastic rubbish bag provided with your prescription and disposed of in a normal waste bin.

Do I need to wipe or wash inside my stoma bag after emptying?

No, however, you should lift the opening upwards to prevent stoma output draining downwards while you are trying to close the opening.

Can I re-use my stoma bag?

No, you cannot re-use your stoma bag, as its adhesive will not be as effective.

Is my stoma bag going to fill up with air and burst?

No, most modern stoma bags have a filter to release air, however, the bag may occasionally fill up with air and begin to leak. You may be able to release excess air by opening the bottom of the stoma bag or unclipping it slightly from the baseplate.

Can I sleep on my abdomen with a stoma?

Though you may not cause any harm to the stoma, your stoma bag may not be able to drain properly or withstand your weight, therefore, it may leak. It is, therefore, better to sleep on your back or side, opposite to the stoma.

How often should I see my stoma nurse?

Initially after surgery your stoma nurse will see you as often as required depending on your individual condition and the local patient pathway used at your hospital. However, it is advisable you are seen at least once a year to review your stoma, ensure you are using the correct stoma products and that your stoma prescription is up to date.

Can I see my stoma nurse if I just need to talk?

Of course, you may wish to speak to your stoma nurse about how your stoma affects your lifestyle or relationships so you do not always have to have a problem with the stoma to be seen by a stoma nurse.

Why should I bring my own stoma supplies when going to the hospital?

There are many stoma products manufacturers with a huge range of products and many hospitals do not have the space to stock all the available options. By bringing your own supplies, you can ensure you have everything you need and the stoma nurse can then order the correct stock if required.

Where should I store my stoma supplies?

You should store your supplies in a cool, dry place and out of the reach of children and pets.

What happens if I run out of stoma supplies?

In the first instance contact your stoma delivery company, pharmacy or prescribing hub. You can also get an emergency supply by contacting your stoma nurse. If you require stock out of working hours, you can contact your local hospital or the ward from where you were discharged and they should be able to provide an emergency supply.

12. Lived experience and patient testimonials

Philip Cox

Sex: Male
Age range at time of surgery: 47–67 years
Diagnosis: Bowel cancer
Was operation emergency or planned: Planned
Type of operation: Open surgery
Type of stoma: Colostomy and urostomy

Life with stoma: I came to terms with living with these two stomas fairly quickly as I was living in great discomfort due to the cancer, so I find the change to my life easier to manage than I envisioned. It seemed strange to begin with but now seems a normal way of life. I find my positive attitude has helped greatly in my situation.

Support received: Stoma nurses at a local hospital and St Mark's Hospital and my wife.

Expectations of surgery: The removal of any risk of cancer remaining. Tough time ahead healing and recovery within 6 months.

Other comments: My healing process from the surgery to remove any cancer and at risk organs has taken longer than expected, but as far as the stomas are concerned they have been fully functional from the beginning.

Francesca Redmore

Sex: Female
Age range at time of surgery: 26–36 years
Diagnosis: Bowel cancer
Was operation emergency or planned: Emergency
Type of operation: Laparoscopic surgery
Type of stoma: Ileostomy

Life with stoma: Life with a stoma is no different from life without a stoma really! At first I had to watch what I ate as too much fibre was a bit risky! But over the course of a couple of months I got back to eating anything I ate previously! I can exercise, socialise, live life as normal with my stoma.

Support received: Stoma care team at St Mark's Hospital – the stoma care nurses were second to none. Simply amazing.

Expectations of surgery: As I had a bowel perforation I just wanted and needed the surgery urgently so did not think too much about it. I felt so relieved when I woke up after the surgery without the pain. The surgery itself was relatively easy to recover from.

Other comments: It took me a couple of weeks to adjust at home to having a stoma to care for, mostly just because it was something different and new, but quite quickly it just became part of me and now I hardly think about it. It helped to look up other young women on social media who also had stomas – this really normalised it all for me, especially seeing models flaunting their bags in holiday pictures. I knew I had nothing to feel embarrassed about and actually felt quite proud!

Robert Lopes de Azevedo-Gilbert

Sex: Male
Age range at time of surgery: Less than 10 years
Diagnosis: Spina bifida, imperforate anus
Was operation emergency or planned: Planned
Type of operation: Open surgery
Type of stoma: Colostomy

Life with stoma: As I have really not known any other lifestyle, it's been terrific, it has not stopped me from doing anything. Yes, there were times I have had to adapt and keep my stoma quiet from employers due to the fact that they would find an excuse not to employ me due to insurance risk. I have done most things when I was younger against advice, as it was still an unknown factor, as most that had a stoma in those days were older generation. I climbed mountains, swimming, scuba diving, horse riding, football, cricket and throwing beer barrels about. One has to learn to adapt to life's inconstancies and do not let it get you down, lift yourself up and learn from life's curved ball.

Support received: At the time there was no stoma nurses or specialist department, that did not come about till the 1960s it was very much learn as you went on. In the beginning there was not even appliances for babies or younger children, all there was were the black rubber bags which at the time were too big for a child. I learnt how to irrigate at the age of four, later came the bags designed for children.

Expectations of surgery: My parents were told to go home and have another child as this one may not make it, well 72 years later I am still around! As a recipient of a stoma and seeing how things have moved forward both in appliances and with surgery advances, which I have been around to see, it has been fantastic, in comparison to how my early years were. This is what I mean by adapting to life's curved balls, today we have support groups, stoma nurses, robotics and laparoscopic surgery and appliances, which we are lucky enough not having to pay for in the UK.

Other comments: I see myself as one of life's fortunate people, from the time of the midwife at home, to being sent to the Children's Hospital in Birmingham and for a very courageous surgeon who, kept my body going until he could perform the stoma operation in July 1948, when the NHS came into fruition. Everything else in life has been a bonus. I have and still having a great life, a few hiccups on the way and no doubt some more to come. Life is what you make of it you can lie down and stop or you do the British thing and get up and brush yourself down and move on, I would not change it for the world, my stoma adapted to my way of life not my stoma controlling me!

Margaret Williams

Sex: Female
Age range at time of surgery: Over 90 years
Diagnosis: Bowel perforation due to diverticulitis
Was operation emergency or planned: Emergency
Type of operation: Open surgery
Type of stoma: Colostomy

Life with stoma: I need to monitor my diet. I am anxious about my stoma bag leaking when I am out and about. This makes me reluctant to attempt a day out.

Support received: I was supported in the stoma care clinic, as well as with visits at home by the community stoma nurses. The community stoma nurses were very helpful in the early days. However, caring for my badly disabled by stroke husband, I was unable to attend the stoma care clinic regularly. There were long gaps between each home visit and many of my phone queries were unanswered, as the stoma care clinic phone was always on answerphone and responses were either delayed or unreturned. An email address for a designated nurse would have been helpful.

Expectations of surgery: Even though I had been warned that the stoma may be permanent I was disappointed when that proved to be the case. I was not given a follow-up clinic appointment with the surgeon after my hospital discharge, as it was Christmas time.

Other comments: The first sight of my stoma was devastating but soon resolved as ward staff was changing my stoma bag. Unfortunately, my stoma nurse went sick and I was not taught how to change my stoma bag for several days. This resulted in a longer stay in hospital until a few days before Christmas. I had a carer at home but at first found caring for my stoma worrying and leakages happened. As I was the main carer for my husband I could not attend the stoma care clinic regularly and for a while had no support. A Macmillan nurse arranged home visits and these were very good but too infrequent.

After my husband died I returned to the stoma care clinic at St Mark's Hospital and my stoma nurse's help and advice were invaluable. My stoma nurse at St Mark's Hospital introduced me to the Inside Out stoma support group taking me there herself, as I would have been anxious going alone. It would have been helpful to have been with the group beforehand and patients need to be advised of this facility before they leave hospital. I learnt a great deal about various devices and seeing a room full of people with the same condition all eager to give advice and help was very supportive.

I was amazed at the outings and foreign holidays they had made. I am 93 years old and do not expect to do these things, but it could be very comforting for younger more active people.

Hazel Pixley

Sex: Female
Age range at time of surgery: Less than 10 years
Diagnosis: Bladder damage due to road traffic accident
Was operation emergency or planned: Planned
Type of operation: Open surgery
Type of stoma: Urostomy

Life with stoma: Difficult as a child. Such things were not spoken about in the 1970s. A lot of school was missed, and I couldn't go to sleepovers or on school trips. Things improved as I grew up, but teenage years were not easy. Now I have the odd leak now and then, but can do most things that others can do. I am married, work full time, go walking at weekends and own/ride a pony.

Support received: Initially from my parents and staff at Great Ormond Street Hospital. There were no stoma care nurses available at that time. My parents joined the Urostomy Association. We had to travel to London for most treatments. Nobody locally knew anything about stomas. We didn't know anybody else who had one.

Expectations of surgery: To become dry, so that teasing/bullying at school would stop.

Other comments: Stomas were definitely a taboo subject in the 1970s, so very few people (even relatives) were told about what I had done. There was little (if any) choice of product and they certainly were not "skin friendly". No stoma care nurses to turn to for assistance. Things have improved a lot now, but there is still further work to do.

Oliver Kaye

Sex: Male
Age range at time of surgery: 10–16 years
Diagnosis: Ulcerative colitis
Was operation emergency or planned: Initially planned then became an emergency
Type of operation: Laparoscopic (keyhole)
Type of stoma: Ileostomy

Life with stoma: The days after my surgery were tough, not only physically but also mentally, accepting my new way of life and actually seeing the stoma for the first time. In hospital I learnt how to clean the area around my stoma and change the bag at first by the stoma nurses, then helped by the nurses and eventually completely on my own which I learnt in just a few days.

When I returned home after my operation, I tried lots of different makes, types of stoma bags that I received samples from the stoma nurses in the hospital. It took me about three weeks to a month to decide on the right bag for me, my choice was guided mainly by the make of the flanges which was easiest for me to empty the bag plus I felt the most comfortable with that bag. For the first month I changed my bag every day to learn how to change my bag and make sure the size was right – as the stoma size can change after surgery. I now change the bag normally every other day and it takes me between 5–10 minutes after I have a shower which is my preferred time to change the bag now.

I thought my diet would change a lot after my surgery. From my surgery I had to very slowly re-integrate food and try the foods to see how my body would react to them. I started with bland foods such as white rice, chicken (no skins) etc. and every week I brought in more foods. I tend to avoid mushrooms, sweetcorn, nuts and seeds completely because they're hard to digest even for the average person. Plus, I peel the fruit skins of fruit, apples, pears etc. I rarely have citrus fruits but I do try to eat fruits mainly bananas, apples and pears but I take multi-vitamin pills to get the extra vitamins in my diet. I started have red meats about 3/4 months' post-op but only have meat from time to time and the same with fast food and I rarely have because it's first unhealthy anyway plus it can be difficult for me to digest. I've had a couple of partial blockages with the stoma so it's so important to chew, chew and chew your foods thoroughly. I also avoid carbonated drinks because it just causes excess gas in the bag which can be inconvenient. Overall I'm happy with my diet, I've been able to gain weight that I lost when I was ill and more to a healthy weight.

I love exercising, playing sports etc. and initially I didn't know if I'll be able to reach the level I was playing pre-diagnosis. However, it was about 3-4 months after my surgery until I did any form of exercise and once the stoma nurses had given me the green light to do so. I began very lightly with trying to tighten my core – tightening my core I actually started before using some exercises recommended and given to me in hospital – which is essential. Then began at very low intensity with walks etc. and every couple of weeks I built up my fitness and strength back up. When I exercise I always wear a stoma support belt and a stoma shield if I'm playing contact sport – football etc. After a long recovery I returned to my football and running in training at first and then playing some matches and now in full fitness I like to say about 7–8 months post-op. Exercising is definitely possible by listening to your body, your stoma nurses and by wearing some form of support for your abdominals. Sport and exercise as I said is a passion of mine that I love so to be able to play again was amazing!

Personally, I think I accepted my stoma relatively quickly because, I was so ill and fed up of being stuck in a hospital bed during a Covid-19 global pandemic, all I wanted was to get better and be healthy and I knew the best chance of this was to have stoma surgery. Before the surgery I reached out to people on Instagram and Facebook and that gave a massive boost that life will get better as I saw these people who are living happy and healthy lives with a bag. This actually inspired me so much to create my own platform @thekidwithabag to raise awareness for people with IBD, stoma bags and invisible illnesses but to also give people some extra inspiration and comfort that life will get better. I made lots of connections with all sorts of people who've had a stoma bag for 10 years or who's having surgery tomorrow. Everyone has their own way of talking about their conditions but social media is a great way to speak to people in similar situations and you can remain anonymous if you want but want to speak to someone who's been through it all.

I had my surgery in June 2020 at St Marks Hospital and my quality of life is so much better, almost normal and I'm grateful to have my life back.

Support received: I received support from St Mark's Hospital's Gastroenterology and Colorectal teams, and paediatric ward. I think my treatment was the best it could've been despite a global pandemic going on. The importance of a good Gastroenterology team is so important.

Expectations of surgery: Initially I was very upset, scared and didn't really know what to expect. I was told it would eliminate my colitis, curing me almost, so should make me better which it did after a long, slow recovery. "Short term pain for long term gain".

Other comments: I'm very grateful to have been treated and supported by St Mark's Hospital who gave my life back. Thank you!

Lee Martin

Sex: Male
Age range at time of surgery: 26–36 years
Diagnosis: Crohn's disease
Was operation emergency or planned: Emergency
Type of operation: Open surgery
Type of stoma: Ileostomy and enterocutaneous fistula

Life with stoma: I have had my stoma for many years so life with it was OK. My stoma bags come pre-cut and I change my stoma bag without any problem and do not need help with it. I was able to go out for a walk or fishing without having to worry. Then I had a complication with bowel obstruction and had to have another surgery. It took long to recover from this operation and I spent many months in hospital, also because I had the fistula where my wound was.

Support received: My mother was helping me. The stoma nurses at St Mark's Hospital showed her how to change my fistula bag and then she was changing my fistula bag when I returned home. I also received support from the stoma care nurses at St Mark's Hospital and my local stoma care nurse.

Expectations of surgery: I was expecting to go back to normal. I was hoping to have my operation to fix the fistula as soon as possible, but it took longer than expected.

Other comments: When I went back home I had to be careful what I eat, because vegetables, fruits and especially onions were bad for my fistula. It took some time before I could go out without my fistula bag leaking. Now I hope to have my operation to fix the fistula soon.

13. Reversal of stoma

Stoma reversal or closure is an operation required to restore bowel continuity. Reversal of your stoma is usually a minor operation compared to your previous surgery and most people are ready to go home 3–7 days after the operation.

Your surgeon will decide when it is safe to have your stoma closed and this usually occurs around 3 months after the formation of the stoma. The length of time to closure depends on your general health, any ongoing treatment you may need and the NHS waiting lists. Unfortunately, stoma reversal is not always priority surgery and some stoma patients are having to wait 6–9 months for this to be done. If you are concerned your stoma has not been closed in a reasonable time and you are not managing, contact your stoma nurse. Occasionally some people may decide to keep their stoma and avoid another operation but this is a personal choice after consultation with their family and surgeon.

Before stoma reversal

Pelvic floor exercises

Pelvic floor exercises tone the muscles in your pelvis, which support your bladder, rectum, anus and reproductive organs and also tone the muscles in and around your anus, to help prevent seepage of stool and wind once your stoma is reversed. There are a variety of exercises that you can do to improve your pelvic floor. These are available online as video tutorials.

> It is important to start doing pelvic floor exercises before your stoma operation and when you have a stoma as the anal sphincters are not being used as much. If you have not been doing pelvic floor exercises before your stoma reversal, you can always start as soon as possible.

You can do pelvic floor exercises by squeezing as tightly as possible the muscles around your back passage and hold for **5 seconds** and then relax the muscles for **10 seconds** between each contraction. Repeat each set at least **10 times** at least **5 times** a day.

Imagine that you are trying to stop yourself from passing wind and urine at the same time to squeeze the muscles around your back passage.

Imagine that you are passing urine and trying to stop the stream of urine. You can try to stop the urine stream just once and only briefly as a way of identifying the right muscles. However, **do not** do this exercise while actually passing urine as this can cause bladder emptying problems.

You can do your pelvic floor exercises while sitting on a chair with your feet on the floor and your legs slightly apart. Once you have mastered this and can isolate the muscles, you should be able to do them in any position, laying, sitting and standing.

Like any other muscle, it will take a few months to see significant improvements.

> ⚠ While doing pelvic floor exercises you should not be squeezing or lifting your buttocks, tensing your abdomen or moving your legs, as this means that you are not doing the exercises correctly.

Distal limb feeding – suitable patients may be offered distal limb feeding before stoma reversal. Distal limb feeding is a form of nutrition administered through the distal (bottom) end of your stoma and into your intestine below. It is believed that distal feeding may reduce your stoma output, provide you with nutrition, water and electrolytes and help reduce or eliminate the need for parenteral nutrition. Additionally, in patients like yourself who are preparing for stoma closure, a small volume of feed is administered through the distal end of your stoma in order to keep the non-functioning distal portion of intestine healthy, help with healing of your intestinal anastomosis and help with your bowel function after closure. Nutrition can be administered as re-infusion of your stoma output or enteral nutrition formula.

You may be considered for distal limb feeding once the date for your stoma reversal operation is booked and contrast studies have excluded any contraindications for distal feeding such as intestinal obstruction, intestinal strictures, anastomotic leaks or sepsis. It is common practice at St Mark's Hospital to be offered distal feeding 6–8 weeks before your stoma closure date and you will continue to administer the feed if you are able to, until you are admitted to hospital for your scheduled stoma reversal operation. A nutrition specialist nurse and a stoma nurse will teach you how to manage your distal feeding regime and arrange all the necessary equipment.

Initially, you may experience complications, such as loose stool and abdominal pain. These are very common side effects of distal feeding. Usually slowing down the administration of the feed will relieve the discomfort. However, if this does not help, contact your specialist nurses who will be able to assist you. As distal feeding is administered through the distal part of your intestine, this will result in increased rectal discharge.

Before your reversal operation, the surgeons may request the following tests to make sure that your operation is a success.

Digital examination – to assess the strength of your anal sphincters (muscles around your back passage). The anal sphincters are responsible for controlling the passage of faeces and wind. If your anal sphincters are weak you may have some incontinence after stoma closure.

Anorectal manometry – to measure how well your anal sphincters and nerves in that area are working. During this test a small catheter with a balloon at the tip will be inserted into the anus and rectum and measurements taken.

X–ray with contrast enema – in order for your surgeon to decide if it is safe to reverse your stoma they need to ensure the surgical joins are healed. A water-soluble enema, containing contrast (dye) is inserted into your back passage and a series of X–rays are taken.

After stoma reversal

Your stoma nurse will usually come to see you on the day after your surgery to discuss topics such as bowel adaptation and retraining, diet and anal skin care and answer any questions you may have. You will be given samples of barrier creams or wipes to prevent anal soreness that may result from opening your bowels more frequently. If your operation is on a Friday, your creams or wipes will be provided by the ward staff.

If you are discharged from hospital over the weekend, a stoma nurse will contact you by telephone to provide advice and support. We will inform your GP or prescribing hub that you have had your stoma reversed and you no longer require a prescription for stoma products. You would no longer require follow-up by your stoma nurse, therefore, you would be discharged from the stoma nursing service.

Dietary advice

After stoma reversal you should be able to return to a normal diet fairly quickly. However, in the first 4–6 weeks after your operation you should follow the same diet you initially followed when you first had your stoma. Refer to the 📖 'immediately post-operation diet' and 📖 'new stoma diet' sections.

Hints and tips following stoma reversal

After stoma reversal it is expected for your bowel function to be quite erratic and unpredictable, with frequent episodes of loose stool or diarrhoea, incontinence, urgency, leakage or constipation. This usually depends on how much of your intestine was removed during your initial surgery, especially the rectum. If a part of your rectum was removed, it will be smaller, therefore, you will need to go to the toilet more often. Your bowel function should settle down in a few weeks, however, sometimes it may take up to a year or even longer for some people.

Loose stool or diarrhoea

- Avoid foods high in fibre, spicy food and fried foods and eat more starchy carbohydrates to thicken your stool. Refer to the 📖 food charts for more information.

- Keep yourself well hydrated to prevent 📖 dehydration by drinking 1.5–2 litres or 8–10 glasses of fluids. Consider adding rehydrating drinks, if diarrhoea persists.

- Medication such as Loperamide can be used to slow down your bowel function but must be taken at least 30 minutes before meals and only with a few sips of water.

- If your diarrhoea is not resolving, your GP may request a stool sample to see if you have an infection such as Clostridium difficile.

Incontinence

Incontinence occurs when you cannot control your bowel movement, leading to partial (soiling) or complete evacuation of loose stool from your anus. After stoma reversal it is normal to experience some soiling, especially at night when the anal sphincter muscles relax but this usually improves in the first few weeks after surgery.

- **Incontinence pad/liners** – may give you a peace of mind and prevent stains on your underwear if you are unable to make it to the toilet on time. Men may benefit from triangular shaped pads which are available in larger supermarkets, rather than regular feminine hygiene products.

- **Absorbent incontinence bed mat/water repellent bed cover** – use to protect your bed in the immediate post stoma reversal period.

- **Keep spare pads and underwear to hand** – many people find it less stressful and feel more prepared for episodes of incontinence if they always carry a small wash bag containing incontinence pads, wet wipes, dry wipes and underwear.

- **Continue to do your pelvic floor exercises** or start to do them, if not previously done.

- **Biofeedback** – if your incontinence persists, speak to your surgeon or GP for a referral to the biofeedback department, where you will be assessed and taught techniques to manage and improve your incontinence.

Urgency or frequency

It is common to experience more urgent signals to empty your bowel or need to go to the toilet more often than usual.

- **Bowel training/urge resistance** – when at home try to delay going to the toilet for as long as you can even if this is only for a couple of minutes. It may be useful keeping yourself distracted by reading a book or watching TV, rather than constantly thinking about going to the toilet.

Anal soreness

Your bottom may get sore if you pass frequent and loose bowel motions.

- Keep the perianal area clean by washing with warm water or water-based, alcohol-free wet wipes and dry well after every bowel motion.
- Use wipes that are suitable for cleaning and moisturising, therefore, you do not need water or barrier cream. Clinell contiplan™ wipes can be purchased online. These can be torn in half to make them more economical.
- Use the shower head attachment or a bidet to wash the area.
- You can use a squirt bottle or travel/portable bidet when out.
- Dry the area gently using soft tissue and avoid rubbing.
- Wear loose cotton underwear.
- Do not use disinfectants or alcohol-based products for cleaning.
- Consider taking medications that help thicken the consistency of your bowel motions.
- Avoid irritating foods such as spicy food and citrus fruit.
- Do not scratch your skin.
- Apply a **thin** layer of barrier cream or a barrier film to your skin to protect the area after every bowel motion and after you have cleaned and dried the area. A mirror may be useful to assist in applying the cream.

Skin protectants available on prescription
• Clinimed® LBF Barrier Cream 100 g tube (code: 3821)
• Pelican Ultra Barrier Cream 50 g tube (code: 130105)
• Brava® Barrier Cream 60 g tube (code: 12000)
• Ilex® Skin Protectant paste – 227 g tub (code: iPT50), 57 g tube (code: iP51)

Skin protectants available over the counter

- Sudocrem®
- Metanium® nappy rash ointment
- Vaseline®

Constipation

- **Keep hydrated** – by drinking 1.5–2 litres or 8–10 glasses of fluids unless advised otherwise due to other medical conditions. Drinks such as coffee or prune juice can help relieve constipation.
- **Regular exercise** – walking is sufficient post stoma closure to keep the bowel moving.
- **Eat plenty of fibre rich foods**, including fruit and vegetables as these foods help prevent and treat constipation.
- **Sit correctly when on the toilet (see diagram)** – as the incorrect position may lead to unsuccessful or incomplete emptying, causing constipation. Try to relax and do not strain. Do not sit on the toilet too long, after 5–10 minutes, you can stand up, massage your abdomen or take a walk, and then sit on toilet again.

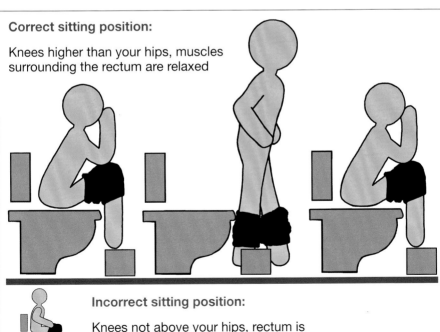

Correct sitting position:

Knees higher than your hips, muscles surrounding the rectum are relaxed

Incorrect sitting position:

Knees not above your hips, rectum is compressed by the surrounding muscles

> If you have had a recent hip surgery, do not lift your knee higher than your hip without consulting your orthopaedic surgeon.

- **Do not delay going to the toilet** – when you feel the need to open your bowels, try not to delay for long periods of time as fluid is reabsorbed causing dry, hardened stool.
- **Laxatives** – if diet and lifestyle changes do not seem to help with constipation, speak to your GP as laxatives may be appropriate.

Post-operative complications

Anastomotic leak

This is an uncommon complication where the join formed during your original operation breaks down and stool begins to leak into your abdominal cavity. This only occurs once your stoma has been reversed. In very rare cases the intestine where the stoma has been closed may leak.

Depending on how extensive the leak is, you may be treated conservatively where you would stop eating and drinking, be given intravenous antibiotics and intravenous fluids and possibly have a drain inserted to remove the collection. If conservative management is not successful, you may require an operation to form a loop stoma to allow healing.

> If you experience fever, abdominal pain, feeling generally unwell, sweating or have an increased heart rate, typically in the first 5–7 days post stoma closure, go to your local emergency department as you may have a leak in your intestine.

Clostridium difficile

Clostridium difficile is an intestinal bacterium that can cause diarrhoea. The infection usually affects people who have recently been treated with antibiotics and can occur within the first month after stoma reversal, though this is not a very common occurrence. Symptoms are diarrhoea, nausea, abdominal cramps and pain, fever and loss of appetite.

If Clostridium difficile is suspected, you will be asked for a stool sample to confirm or exclude the infection. Additionally, you may need an abdominal scan and blood tests to confirm or exclude a leak in the intestine, as Clostridium difficile may mimic symptoms of a leak. If Clostridium difficile is confirmed, you will need to isolate in a single room in order to prevent infection spreading to other people and will have to limit visitors. You should also use a separate bathroom. It is also very important to wash your hands regularly with soap and water. You will be given oral antibiotics and then another stool sample taken to confirm the infection has been treated.

Hernia

During stoma reversal your surgeon needs to cut through your abdominal muscles again, which means that you are at risk of developing a hernia.

Wound infection

In order to prevent the surface of the stoma closure site healing before the tissue below, the wound may be left slightly open to allow granulation tissue to form. The wound may take slightly longer to heal and care should be taken to change the dressings regularly to prevent a wound infection. You should see the practice nurse at your GP surgery if you are concerned that healing is slow or that you have developed an infection.

Low anterior resection syndrome (LARS)

LARS usually presents as a combination of the following symptoms that can drastically effect your quality of life after stoma closure.

- frequency or urgency of bowel movements
- incomplete emptying and opening your bowels multiple times
- faecal incontinence with an inability to control your bowel movements
- constipation lasting a few days, followed by diarrhoea
- increased wind
- abdominal pain
- anal skin excoriation

The common causes are a smaller rectum after the removal of part of your rectum, or a weakness or damage to the anal sphincter muscles after chemotherapy, radiotherapy or surgery.

Persistent symptoms can be managed by:

- **Neuromuscular electrical stimulation of the pelvic floor (NMES)** – aims to strengthen your anal sphincter muscles with the use of a small device and electrodes attached to your pelvic floor muscles. The device sends electrical impulses to your muscles, which helps them contract and strengthen. A specialist nurse will teach you how to use NMES but it may take several months to notice any benefit.
- **Sacral nerve stimulation (SNS)** – is an implant placed under your skin above the buttock. The SNS is the size of a £2 coin and its battery lasts approximately 5 years. The SNS sends messages to your pelvic floor

muscles helping manage faecal continence by retraining the muscles.

- **Transanal irrigation** – is a procedure to help regulate the passage of stool. Approximately 500–1000 ml of lukewarm water (37°C degree) is inserted into your back passage using a special soft cone or a catheter. The water then distends your intestine causing peristalsis or wave-like motions that expel the stool and wind (flatus) from your intestine. While the success of transanal irrigation is purely individual, research suggests very promising results with significantly reduced bowel motions after starting transanal irrigation.

 Once your stoma has been reversed you can contact your local stoma nurse or charitable organisations, such as **Jacob's Well Appeal**, to arrange for your stoma products to be collected for donation to countries who cannot afford these products.

Appendices

1. St Mark's Hospital stoma patient pathway

OUTPATIENTS: Pre-operation counselling

- Face-to-face or telephone or virtual consultation
- Stoma siting (if appropriate)
- Provide stoma practice kit and Stoma Care Book

IN HOSPITAL: Inpatient stoma care

- Stoma siting (if not yet sited)
- Stoma teaching – daily/twice daily
- Stoma complications prevention/management
- Psycho-social support, dietary and lifestyle advice

0–10 DAYS POST-DISCHARGE: Local patients

- Provide one week of stoma products
- Register patient with Harrow Appliance Prescription Service (HAPS)
- Daily telephone support via Secure Start™
- 1 x face-to-face or telephone or virtual follow-up or home visit (for housebound patients)
  - Clinical appliance use and prescription review
  - Stoma complications prevention/management
  - Psycho-social support, dietary and lifestyle advice

0–10 DAYS POST-DISCHARGE: Tertiary patients

- Provide two weeks of stoma products
- Register with a DAC
- Refer to local stoma nurse
- Discharge from St Mark's Hospital stoma care service

11–30 DAYS POST-DISCHARGE: Routine follow-up

- 1 x face-to-face or telephone or virtual follow-up or home visit (for housebound patients)
  - Clinical appliance use and prescription review
  - Stoma complications prevention/management
  - Psycho-social support, dietary and lifestyle advice

MONTH 3 POST-DISCHARGE: Routine follow-up and stoma reversal counselling

- 1 x face-to-face or telephone or virtual follow-up or home visit (for housebound patients)
  - Clinical appliance use and prescription review
  - Stoma complications prevention/management
  - Psycho-social support, dietary and lifestyle advice
- 1 x telephone consultation via Secure Start™
- Discuss stoma reversal (if appropriate)
  - Discuss distal feeding (if appropriate)

MONTH 12 POST-DISCHARGE: long term follow-up

- 1 x face-to-face or telephone or virtual follow-up or home visit (for housebound patients)
  - Clinical appliance use and prescription review
  - Stoma complications prevention/management
  - Psycho-social support, dietary and lifestyle advice
- 1 x telephone consultation via Secure Start™
- Arrange annual follow-up appointment

PATIENT UNDERGOING STOMA REVERSAL

- Inpatient support
  - Discuss bowel adaptation and retraining
  - Discuss anal skin care and provide barrier cream
  - Reiterate importance of pelvic floor exercises
  - Psycho-social support, dietary and lifestyle advice
  - Reiterate hernia prevention
  - Provide written information
  - Advise to contact St Mark's Hospital surgical team if signs and symptoms of LARS or incontinence
- Discharge from stoma care
  - Inform DAC & GP that patient will no longer require stoma products
  - Inform local stoma nurses that patient has had their stoma reversed

2. St Mark's Hospital stoma patient meal plan examples

Meal plan examples up to 6 weeks after stoma formation:

Patient meal plan advice

- Choose cooking methods such as slow and pressure cooking.
- If your appetite is poor, use snacks as main meal rather than not eating.
- If you are vegan/vegetarian replace meat/poultry with soy-based or other meat substitutes.
- Try mixing and matching the meals so you can have a wider variety of choices.

Breakfast

- Scrambled/poached egg and white toast
- Rice Krispies®/corn flakes/Coco Pops® with milk
- Porridge and peeled tinned fruit (no pineapple)
- Plain yogurt and banana (ripe)
- Cream cheese and smoked salmon on a plain bagel
- Crêpe with chocolate spread
- Smooth peanut butter and white toast
- Greek yogurt with honey and banana
- Pancakes and banana slices (ripe)
- Plain scone with butter and smooth jam
- Scrambled/poached egg and ham muffin
- Grilled egg and cheese sandwich (white bread)
- Soft-boiled eggs and white toast and avocado
- White bread/toast with butter and honey/smooth jam
- Waffles with honey and fruit juice (no pulp)
- Plain omelette and croissant

Lunch and dinner

- Skinless chicken/turkey breast/thigh in gravy with white rice and well-cooked peeled courgettes
- Pasta with grated cheese, blended tomato sauce and minced meat/soya mince
- Fish and mashed potatoes

- Jacket potato (no skin) with butter and cheese
- Quiche Lorraine
- Shepherd's pie (no onions, peas, corn, celery)
- Skinless chicken/tender pork with noodles
- Well-cooked tender rosemary pork and mashed potatoes with gravy
- Chicken wrap (white) with grilled courgettes/bell peppers (no skin)
- Creamy pasta with poultry/fish/slow-cooked meat
- Slow-cooked tender lamb with mint and well-cooked peeled carrots and potatoes
- Chicken mild curry (e.g. Korma) with white rice
- Peeled grilled aubergine slices with feta cheese
- Chicken noodle soup
- Pesto and cheese tortellini
- Baked fish fingers and well-cooked peeled carrots
- Baked scotch egg and mashed potatoes
- Fish pie and mushy peas
- Spaghetti bolognese
- Roasted tender pork and white rice
- Slow-cooked tender beef/pork/lamb stew
- Tuna mayonnaise sandwich (white bread)
- Ham/chicken and cheese sandwich (white bread)
- Cream of tomato/potato/butternut squash soup
- Tofu burger with mashed avocado
- Pizza Margherita
- Fish and peeled baby potatoes and broccoli florets (no stalks)
- Soy mince and vegetable lasagne (no skin)
- Slow-cooked tender lamb and courgette risotto
- Slow-cooked tender beef casserole
- Well-cooked tender beef/pork and roasted potatoes
- Stuffed sweet peppers with minced meat and rice
- Macaroni and cheese and cauliflower florets (no stalks)
- Pasta with roasted butternut squash and feta cheese
- Steamed pork dumplings with soy sauce
- Gnocchi with pesto and grated cheese

Dessert or snacks

- Rice/tapioca pudding
- Ice cream/frozen yogurt (no nuts/fruit)
- Smooth yogurt (no nuts/fruit)
- Banana
- Plain cakes
- Crisps
- Cottage cheese and plain crackers (no nuts)
- Custard
- Apple pie and custard
- Rice/corn cakes and cheese/avocado/chocolate spread
- Cheese and plain biscuits/crackers (no nuts/fruit)
- Marshmallows
- Jelly babies
- Apple sauce and cottage cheese
- Smooth jelly
- Breadsticks and ham
- Sea-salted pretzels
- White chocolate
- Watermelon slices (no seeds)
- Peeled apple slices with smooth peanut butter
- Peeled tinned fruit (no pineapple)

3. St Mark's Hospital guide to managing stoma obstruction

SIGNS AND SYMPTOMS

- Stoma output reduced
- Thin, watery output
- Output has a different colour
- Output has an offensive smell
- Bloated abdomen
- Abdominal cramping
- Pain around stoma

ACTIONS TO BE TAKEN

- Stop eating
- Drink fluids only
- Quickly drink 1–2 glasses of water to flush out possible obstruction
- Massage abdomen and around stoma
- Lay down with knees to chest or try side to side rolling to move obstruction
- Do light exercise such as walking
- Have a warm bath
- Use a hot water bottle to relax your abdomen and relieve pain
- Cut the opening of stoma baseplate slightly larger than usual, if the stoma is swollen
- Do not take laxatives

SIGNS AND SYMPTOMS

- Stoma stops working
- Increased abdominal cramping and pain
- Abdomen looks more bloated
- Nausea
- Vomiting

ACTIONS TO BE TAKEN

- Stop drinking
- Go to the emergency department
- Take your stoma wash bag with you

EMERGENCY DEPARTMENT MANAGEMENT

ACTIONS TO BE TAKEN

- Nil by mouth
- Nasal gastric tube inserted
- Intravenous fluids
- Catheter in stoma
- Pain management
- CT scan/X–ray
- Ward care for observation
- Surgery (only if appropriate)

4. St Mark's Hospital guide to managing high output stoma

Managing high output stoma greater than 1500 ml:

DETERMINE CAUSE

- Have you had any food/drinks that may have upset your stomach or that you do not usually tolerate well?
- Have you had a meal which was eaten raw or had under-cooked food?
- Have you taken antibiotics, laxatives or medications that may cause diarrhoea as a side effect?
- Have you travelled abroad recently and picked up an infection?
- Do you feel generally unwell?

INITIAL MANAGEMENT

- Monitor fluid intake and stoma output accurately
- Stop eating **high fibre** and **spicy** foods
- Add **extra salt** to your meals
- Drink **rehydration drinks** such as **E–Mix solution/ Dioralyte™** – 1 litre/24 hours
- **Restrict hypotonic fluids** to 0.5–1 litre/24 hours (tea, coffee, water, juice, squash, etc.) and **hypertonic fluids** (juice, fizzy drinks, Ensure®)
- Eat foods **rich in potassium** – bananas, smooth peanut butter, potatoes, oranges
- Eat foods **rich in salt** – crackers and savoury biscuits (no seeds/nuts), crisps, cheese
- Eat **output thickening** food – bananas, white rice, apple sauce, white toast, mashed potatoes, marshmallows, tapioca pudding
- Take **Loperamide** as instructed, 30 minutes before meals and before bed
- Take **Codeine Phosphate** as instructed
- Take **anti-secretory medication** as instructed

FURTHER MANAGEMENT

IF NO IMPROVEMENT WITHIN 48–72 HOURS

Contact you stoma nurse or go to your local emergency department if your high output persist after 48–72 hours and you feel unwell or dehydrated.

ST MARK'S E–MIX SOLUTION

- 6 level teaspoons of Glucose powder – 20 grams.
- 1 level teaspoon of Sodium Chloride (table salt) – 3.5 grams.
- Half a heaped teaspoon of Sodium Bicarbonate (baking soda) – 2.5 grams.

Dissolve all the ingredients in 1 litre of water and sip over 24 hours. You can add a tiny splash of squash for a better taste or keep the solution refrigerated. **Do not add ice** as this dilutes the solution. The ingredients can be bought from the chemist or the supermarket.

DIORALYTE™

- Mix 10 sachets in 1 litre of water.
- Alternatively, you can mix 2 sachets in a 200 ml glass of water, 5 times a day.

Drink the solution slowly over 24 hours. You can buy Dioralyte™ from the chemist or the supermarket.

Dioralyte™ is high in potassium therefore it needs to be taken with caution.

5. St Mark's Hospital troubleshooting guide for colostomy irrigation

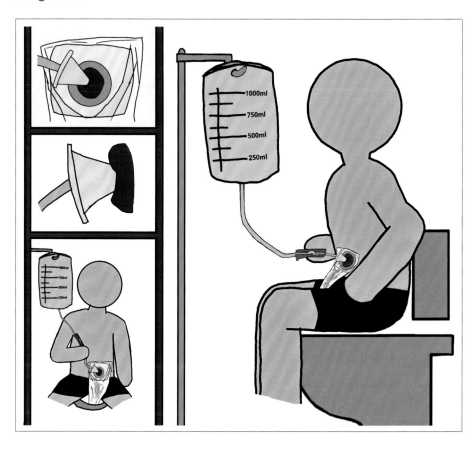

Abdominal cramping during irrigation	
Cause	**Solution**
Water is too hot or cold	• Stop irrigation and wait for the cramps to resolve • Take deep breaths and massage your abdomen • Check the temperature of the water • If the water is too hot/cold, discard water and refill container/bag with lukewarm water (37°C)
Introducing water into your colostomy too quickly	• Stop irrigation and wait for cramps to resolve • Take deep breaths and massage abdomen • Slow down the water flow rate

Feeling faint/lightheaded or nauseated during irrigation	
Cause	**Solution**
Vasovagal reaction caused by excessive distention of the colon	• Stop irrigation and only continue when sensation is gone • Slow down water flow rate • Check water temperature is still at 37°C • Decrease the amount of water for irrigation • Consult stoma nurse if problem persists

Stoma is active between irrigations	
Cause	**Solution**
Incorrect irrigation water amount	• Increase irrigation water if solid/semi formed stoma output present • Reduce amount of irrigation water if liquid output present
Too much time between irrigations	• Irrigate daily instead of every other day • Irrigate your stoma at the same time of day • Irrigate with half the water and allow colon to empty Then insert the rest of the water after a short break

Water leaking around stoma	
Cause	**Solution**
Stoma cone not inserted correctly	• Try changing the angle of the cone • Ensure you are holding the cone securely in place • Slow down water flow rate
Thick output obstructing the cone	• Remove the cone, inspect it for stoma output and rinse if needed • Consider drinking more fluid and staying hydrated

Difficulty inserting the stoma cone	
Cause	**Solution**
Stoma cone not angled in the right direction	• Gently insert a lubricated finger into the colostomy and identify the correct direction of your colon • Try changing your position, lean forwards or stand • Try relaxing and not tensing your abdominal muscles • You may have developed a stoma stricture, prolapse or hernia therefore contact your stoma nurse

Water put in stoma does not come out	
Cause	**Solution**
Inadequate irrigation water	• Increase irrigation water amount up to 1000 ml – do not exceed 1000 ml without consulting your stoma nurse
Dehydration – intestine absorbing irrigation water	• Keep yourself hydrated • Try drinking 1–2 glasses of water or a hot drink before irrigation • Reduce alcohol or caffeine consumption which may lead to dehydration
Parastomal hernia	• Bulging or pain around your stoma when inserting the water may mean you have a parastomal hernia. Contact your stoma nurse, as irrigation may no longer be suitable for you

Bleeding from stoma	
Cause	**Solution**
Trauma during cone insertion	• Insert the cone gently and do not force it if you feel any resistance • Digitate stoma and identify correct direction of colon • Use more lubricating gel

Glossary

- **Abdomen** – the part of your body between your chest and the top of your hips, also known as the 'tummy' or 'belly'
- **Abnormal** – not normal or naturally occurring
- **Absorb** – the process where your body soaks up fluids, food and medications
- **Accessible toilet** – a bigger toilet designed for people with wheelchairs, mobility difficulties, people with a stoma or bowel and bladder problems
- **Accessory** – product used with stoma bag (e.g. adhesive remover spray; rings; etc.)
- **Acid–base balance** – mechanisms used by your body to keep its fluids to a certain pH so it can function properly
- **Adhesions** – scars within your abdomen which may cause the intestine to stick to other organs or itself
- **Administer** – to be given something such as medications
- **Anastomosis** –the joining of two separate parts of tube-like organs, for example blood vessels or intestines
- **Anus** – the last part of your digestive system, also known as the 'back passage'
- **Appliance** – another word used for stoma bag and pouching system
- **Biopsy** – a sample of tissue taken for laboratory tests
- **Bowel preparation** – cleansing medication that help you empty your bowels completely usually before surgery or medical examination and may cause diarrhoea
- **Chronic** – illness or condition which you have had for a long time
- **Colon** – part of your digestive system also known as the large intestine
- **Contaminate** – to make something unclean
- **DAC** – Dispensing Appliance Contractor. These are the companies that deliver your stoma products.
- **Deficiency** – when your body lacks important electrolytes, vitamins or minerals
- **Digest** – to break down food into smaller pieces that the body can use
- **Digestive enzymes** – are produced by your mouth, stomach, pancreas and small intestine to help break down food and fluids
- **Distal washout** – usually done in people with a loop stoma to help clear the downstream part of intestine before a procedure or help clear up any built up mucus
- **Diuretic drinks** – drinks that increase the amount of urine your body produces making you lose more fluids and electrolytes
- **Divert** – to change direction
- **Dusky** – dark red, brown or grey colour
- **Dysplasia** – abnormal growth of cells in organs often linked to

precancerous growth

- **Electrolytes** – elements in your blood that help keep your body functioning properly (e.g. salt; potassium; magnesium; calcium)
- **Eliminate/expel/evacuate** – to remove something out of your body
- **Endoscopy** – a procedure used to observe an internal organ or tissue by using a long, thin tube inserted directly into the mouth, anus or stoma
- **Enteral feed/enteral nutrition formula** – additional nutrition given to you through a tube going into your stomach or intestine
- **Faeces/faecal matter** – the waste product of digestion also known as 'stool' or 'poo'
- **Fashion** – to surgically make or create something
- **Flaccid** – flabby or loose
- **Fluids** – any types of drinks or liquid
- **Fluid overload** – is a condition where too much fluid builds up in your body causing swelling, especially immediately after surgery or if you have heart problems
- **Fortified foods** – foods with added electrolytes, vitamins and minerals (example milk with added vitamin D or bread with added vitamin B_{12})
- **Haemoserous fluid** – light, pink liquid mixed with blood, commonly produced by your stoma immediately after operation
- **Hollow organ** – a tube-like organ, which has walls on the outside and is empty on the inside
- **Hypertonic fluids** – types of fluids which bring water together with salt into your intestine which can be lost through your stoma
- **Hypotonic fluids** – types of fluids which bring salt into your intestine which can be lost through your stoma
- **Incision** – a surgical cut made during an operation
- **Incorporate** – to include something into something else
- **Intravenous fluids** – fluids given directly into your vein especially if you are dehydrated or cannot eat and drink
- **Ischaemia** – occurs when the blood supply to an organ or tissue is reduced or stopped, causing tissue death. When ischaemia occurs, the organ or tissue becomes **ischaemic**
- **Isotonic fluids** – types of fluids which help keep you hydrated, as they are high in salt and help the body keep fluid and reduce losses through the stoma
- **Low-residue diet** – foods which leave minimal 'residue' of undigested food after digestion. They are **easy to digest** and **low on fibre** (e.g. tender meats; fish and poultry without skin; eggs; white pasta/bread/rice; peeled and well-cooked soft/mashed vegetables and fruits, etc.)
- **Metabolise** – the process of turning food and other nutrients, into energy, new cells and waste products

- **Minerals** – vital elements your body needs in small quantities in order to function and develop properly
- **Mucosa** – the lining of your stoma which appears red and moist
- **Mucus** – a natural lubricant produced by your intestine, which is usually a clear or white liquid or may be quite thick and sticky
- **Nausea** – a general feeling of discomfort felt before you vomit
- **Necrosis** – premature cell death caused by injury, infection, lack of blood supply. When necrosis occurs, a tissue becomes **necrotic**
- **Nutrients** – important food elements that help your body function properly
- **Obstruction** – when something blocks your stoma or intestine so it does not empty properly
- **Oedematous** – term used to describe body tissue with an excessive build-up of fluids causing swelling
- **Ooze** – when a liquid discharge is coming out (**oozing**) from an opening in your body
- **Oral/orally** – when food, drinks or medications are taken by mouth
- **Output** – faecal or urine waste produced by your stoma
- **Parastomal hernia** – bulging of your intestine under the stoma and peristomal skin
- **Parenteral nutrition** – nutrition given directly into your blood stream through a large vein
- **Pelvic region/pelvis** – this is the lower end of your body, just under your belly button and where organs, such as your bladder, rectum and reproductive organs are found
- **Penetrate** – to go into or through something
- **Perforation** – a hole/tear in your intestine caused by severe inflammation, tumour growth, trauma or sometimes during endoscopy or surgical investigations
- **Perineal area/perineum** – the skin and surrounding area near your bottom or back passage
- **Peristomal skin** – the skin surrounding your stoma
- **Precancerous** – abnormal cell growth that may increase the risk of cancer
- **Pre-existing medical condition** – any condition you've been diagnosed with in the past (e.g. asthma; diabetes; heart problems; allergies, etc.)
- **Pulses** – these are type of foods that include all beans, lentils, peas, etc.
- **Rectum** – is part of your large intestine, its main function is to store waste products until you are able to open your bowels
- **Refashion** – to re-shape or change something (e.g. refashion a stoma)
- **Relapse** – to begin experiencing signs and symptoms of a disease after a period without illness
- **Remission** – signs and symptoms of a disease are less severe or have

disappeared completely

- **Resection** – removal of part or all of an organ
- **Retract** – drop or go below
- **Stricture** – when your intestine or stoma narrows making it more difficult for waste to pass through
- **Supplements** – these can be tablets, injections, patches or sprays taken to support your body if you do not receive enough electrolytes, vitamins and minerals
- **Synthesis** – the process during which your body produces vital elements (e.g. Vitamin K; vitamin B, etc.)
- **Vitamins** – vital elements your body needs in small quantities in order to function and develop properly
- **Waste product** – materials your body does not need and are removed in urine and faeces

References

1. British Healthcare Trades Association (BHTA 2021). Sponsored vs non-sponsored - Analysis of selected CCG data based on contract changes over last 4 years. June 2020.

2. Lister, S., Hofland, J., Grafton, H. The Royal Marsden Manual of Clinical Nursing Procedures. Chapter 6: Elimination. Wiley-Blackwell; 10th Edition, Professional edition 30 April 2020, p. 255.